The Belly Fat Prognosis

Transform Your Body & Mind to Lose Weight and Keep It Off for a Younger, Healthier You!

Kelly Kam

© **Copyright 2024 - All rights reserved.**

The content contained within this book may not be reproduced, duplicated or transmitted without direct written permission from the author or the publisher.

Under no circumstances will any blame or legal responsibility be held against the publisher, or author, for any damages, reparation, or monetary loss due to the information contained within this book, either directly or indirectly.

Legal Notice:

This book is copyright protected. It is only for personal use. You cannot amend, distribute, sell, use, quote or paraphrase any part, or the content within this book, without the consent of the author or publisher.

Disclaimer Notice:

Please note the information contained within this document is for educational and entertainment purposes only. All effort has been executed to present accurate, up to date, reliable, complete information. No warranties of any kind are declared or implied. Readers acknowledge that the author is not engaged in the rendering of legal, financial, medical or professional advice. The content within this book has been derived from various sources. Please consult a licensed professional before attempting any techniques outlined in this book.

By reading this document, the reader agrees that under no circumstances is the author responsible for any losses, direct or indirect, that are incurred as a result of the use of the information contained within this document, including, but not limited to, errors, omissions, or inaccuracies.

Table of Contents

INTRODUCTION 1

Chapter 1: The Belly Fat Dilemma—Understanding the Complexity and Challenges........ 3
Chapter 2: Why This Book? A Comprehensive Guide to a Healthier You...................... 5

PART I: UNDERSTANDING BELLY FAT 7

Chapter 3: What Is Belly Fat? An In-Depth Examination................................. 9
Chapter 4: The Science Behind Belly Fat—Exploring the Biological Factors............... 13
Chapter 5: The Role of Genetics in Accumulating Belly Fat..................................... 15
Chapter 6: Why Is Losing Belly Fat So Hard? Unravelling the Mystery..................... 17
Chapter 7: Obesity Epidemic—A Global Health Crisis.. 21

PART II: IMPLICATION OF EXCESSIVE BELLY FAT 23

Chapter 8: Diseases Indicated by an Increased Waistline.. 25
Chapter 9: The Metabolic Menace.. 29
The Invisible Threat..29
Unravelling the Solution...30
Chapter 10: How Belly Fat Affects Your Heart, Liver, and Other Organs.................. 31
Chapter 11: Mental Health Concerns Related to Obesity.. 35

PART III: ANALYSING TRIGGERS FOR DEVELOPING VISCERAL FAT...........39

Chapter 12: Sedentary Lifestyle and Its Effects on Body Weight.............................. 41
The Science Behind Sedentarism.. 41
Chapter 13: Stress Eating and Emotional Overeating—Unhealthy Coping Mechanisms 43
Chapter 14: Impact of Alcohol, Smoking, and Drug Use on Weight Gain................. 47
Chapter 15: Sleep Deprivation and Its Correlation With Obesity............................. 51

PART IV: DIETARY CONSIDERATIONS FOR REDUCING ABDOMINAL BULGE........55

Chapter 16: Food Habits That Lead to Excess Pounds.. 57
Chapter 17: Superfood Compounds That Fight Against Obesity; Spotlight on Anthocyanin..61
Power of Anthocyanin... 63
Chapter 18: Meal Planning Strategies for Sustainable Weight Loss......................... 67

PART V: EXERCISE ESSENTIALS IN FIGHTING FLAB... 71

Chapter 19: Exercise Basics for Burning Calories Effectively................................... 73
Chapter 20: Belly Battles—Specific Exercises for Abdominal Reduction................... 77
Chapter 21: How Much Physical Activity Do You Really Need?............................... 81

PART VI: BEHAVIOURAL CHANGES FOR LONG-TERM SUCCESS..................... 83

Chapter 22: Mindful Eating Techniques to Control Caloric Intake........................... 85
Chapter 23: Building Resilience Towards Food Cravings.. 89
Chapter 24: Motivation Maintenance Strategies for Consistent Efforts....................93

PART VII: LIVING YOUNG & AGING HEALTHY 95
Chapter 25: Anti-Ageing Secrets and Belly Fat—The Undeniable Connection 97
Chapter 26: How to Achieve a Healthy Lifestyle for Longevity 101
Chapter 27: Importance of Regular Health Check-Ups 105

PART VIII: MANAGING WEIGHT IN DIFFERENT LIFE STAGES 107
Chapter 28: Losing Baby Weight—Post-Pregnancy Waistline Woes 109
Chapter 29: Dealing With Midlife Metabolism Slowdown 111
If Things Are Extra Bad? *114*
Chapter 30: Elderly and Obesity—Special Considerations 115

PART IX: OVERCOMING OBSTACLES IN YOUR FITNESS JOURNEY 119
Chapter 31: Plateauing—When the Scale Doesn't Budge Anymore 121
Chapter 32: Bouncing Back From Failures and Setbacks 125
Chapter 33: Preparing for Unexpected Changes and Challenges 127

CONCLUSION 131
Chapter 34: Making Peace With Your Body—Self-Love and Acceptance 133
Chapter 35: Maintaining the Momentum—Creating a Lifelong Plan for Health 135

FOOD PORTIONS: A QUICK GUIDE 139
Proteins 140
Carbohydrates 141
Fruits and Vegetables 142

GLOSSARY 145

REFERENCES 149

ABOUT THE AUTHOR 163

Introduction

Chapter 1:
The Belly Fat Dilemma—Understanding the Complexity and Challenges

Belly fat—the two words evoke an array of emotions ranging from frustration to despair. What is belly fat? Why do we get it? And why is losing it so difficult? These questions have haunted many for ages but are unfortunately often ignored or answered incorrectly. Allow me to take you on a journey into the enigmatic world of belly fat. Before we embark, let us stow away any preconceived notions about this seemingly innocuous substance. What gets in the way of tackling a problem is not what we do not know; rather, it is what we think we know for sure but is just not so!

The first step towards solving any problem is to understand it. Let us start by defining belly fat. A burgeoning waistline is often a combination of a layer of fat accumulating just beneath the skin, called subcutaneous fat, and deep abdominal fat surrounding our organs, scientifically known as visceral fat (*Belly Fat in Women*, 2023). Visceral fat is a type of fat (adipose) tissue with a high density of blood vessels that releases hormones and responds to neurotransmitters. This makes it metabolically more active and stubbornly resistant to traditional weight-loss efforts. Increased visceral fat is also linked with decreased insulin sensitivity, making it difficult to lose this type of fat (Liu et al., 2017; Quaglia, 2021). This is one of the main reasons why losing abdominal fat can seem like climbing Mount Everest without an oxygen tank. But here comes the plot twist. Belly fat is not just an aesthetic nuisance—it is also a potential harbinger of various health risks like diabetes, heart disease, and certain cancers (*Abdominal Fat*, 2019). Visceral fat is also linked with the incidence of high blood pressure and dementia (Collins, 2023).

Why do we accumulate belly fat? The answer lies largely in today's sedentary lifestyles and high-calorie food intake. In simple terms: too much sitting and eating without burning those calories. Losing that belly fat may seem arduous if you do not know where to start or what to do. Few exercises can target that stubborn belly fat specifically. Even seemingly lean individuals accumulate unhealthy belly fat if they are physically inactive (Collins, 2023). When trying to lose belly fat, keep in mind that you are not at war with your body. Your body is not your enemy here—misunderstanding is. So, then, how do we fight this battle? The answer is knowledge—specifically, understanding how your body works and interacts with food, exercise, sleep patterns, etc.—thereby adopting a sustainable lifestyle change instead of quick fixes or fad diets. Losing abdominal fat is a slow process that requires patience and consistent effort. It is not about adopting a diet but about a lifestyle change that can help you live younger, healthier, and happier.

Key Takeaways

- Belly fat, aka visceral fat, is different from subcutaneous fat.
- It is metabolically active, making it hard to lose.
- It is associated with various health risks.
- Understanding its nature and adopting healthy lifestyle changes instead of a diet is the key to losing it.

Chapter 2:

Why This Book? A Comprehensive Guide to a Healthier You

> *Health is like money, we never have a true idea of its value until we lose it.*
>
> -Josh Billings

This book is not about losing weight for vanity's sake. It is not about fitting into that little black dress or those skinny jeans that have been gathering dust in your wardrobe. It is definitely not about looking good at the beach (although these could be welcomed side effects.). This book is about something far more significant—your health and your life.

Let me paint you a picture. Imagine an enemy silently creeping up on you—slowly but surely wrapping its insidious tendrils around your organs, choking their functionality, and robbing them of vitality. This is what belly fat does to your body. As discussed before, belly fat is more than just an aesthetic issue; it is a silent killer linked to several chronic diseases. So, why is all this discussion regarding belly fat alone? Well, not all fats are created equal. The fat sitting on our hips might make us cringe when we look in the mirror, but it poses a lesser threat when compared to the one nestling deep within our abdomen and padding our organs. Studies describe visceral fat as an endocrine organ that secretes hormones and harmful substances capable of triggering inflammation—a root cause of many chronic and metabolic disorders (*Abdominal Fat*, 2019).

As we traverse through the subsequent chapters of this book, we will explore the intricacies of belly fat—its causes, consequences, and, most importantly, how best to banish it—all while explaining the science in an easy and digestible way. Now, I can almost see some eyes glazing over at the thought of scientific jargon and complex terminologies. Fear not. This journey is designed to be like a leisurely walk in a park, with simple language, short paragraphs, a little sprinkle of humour, and easy-to-understand metaphors. Before you know it, you will be armed with advanced tips on tackling stubborn belly fat, even when the problem seems insurmountable. You will learn why belly fat tends to be so stubborn (spoiler alert: It has more to do with hormones than willpower). You will discover how to combat this through simple changes in your diet and lifestyle. The key is to understand the adversary and work smarter—not harder.

Exercise plays a part in losing stubborn belly fat, but it does not necessarily imply hours on the treadmill (unless, of course, that is your thing.). We will introduce fun ways to stay active and burn calories without even realising you are doing it. But what if the problem seems impossible to overcome? What if diets have failed and gym memberships have been wasted? Do not worry. We have you covered. This book provides life-changing recommendations and alternative solutions for those needing that little extra bit of help. You will understand why some methods do not work while others do—and what to do instead.

Let us embark on this exploration together—hand in hand—towards understanding the mystery of belly fat and discovering ways to conquer it once and for all. However, remember that the road to victory is not always smooth or straight—it has its ups and downs—but each step forward brings us closer to our goal. By the end of this journey, you will have gained several "ah-ha" moments as you understand why certain problems occur in the first place, how best to solve them, and why these solutions work.

Key Takeaways

- Belly fat is more dangerous than other types of body fat.
- Lifestyle habits play a significant role in accumulating belly fat.
- Simple changes in diet and lifestyle can help combat this issue.
- Advanced tips and choices are available for those needing extra help.

Part I:

Understanding Belly Fat

Chapter 3:
What Is Belly Fat? An In-Depth Examination

For anybody who is not a complete stranger to the world of health and fitness, one term that cannot be ignored is "belly fat." It is not just a cosmetic concern; it is also linked with various health issues. So, what exactly is belly fat? And why does it matter? Let us look into this in detail.

Belly fat—medically referred to as visceral fat—is the excess abdominal fat surrounding your organs. Unlike subcutaneous fat, which lies under your skin, this stubborn deposit of extra pounds resides deep within your body and poses serious threats to your well-being. Visceral fat (also referred to as intra-abdominal fat) accounts for about one-tenth of total belly fat. It accumulates beneath the abdominal wall in the spaces around the intestines, liver, and other organs (*Taking Aim*, 2024). An easy way to differentiate between subcutaneous and visceral fat is to look at the area where the fat is accumulated. If the fat is concentrated around the hips and lower body, giving you a pear shape, and can be easily pinched with your fingers, it is subcutaneous fat. Fat around the midsection and waist tends to be visceral, and it gives you an apple-shaped body (*Abdominal Fat*, 2019). At normal levels, visceral fat provides cushioning and insulation to organs. It also stores energy and secretes hormones and other molecules that help in endocrinological signalling (Shuster et al., 2012). The reason losing belly fat feels like an uphill battle has its roots in our physiology. Belly fats have more alpha-receptors than beta-receptors, which inhibit the breakdown of fats (Lopes et al., 2016). In simple terms, they are designed to stay put.

You might wonder why we accumulate belly fat in the first place. The culprits are many—unhealthy eating habits, a sedentary lifestyle, and stress being some of them. But an interesting fact here is our evolutionary history. Our ancestors needed these extra calories for survival during times of famine—a trait not so useful in today's age of abundance. Our bodies are programmed for survival, dating back to caveman days when food was scarce; thus, when excess calories enter our system, they get stored as 'energy reserves', aka fats. An individual's genetic makeup also impacts where fat gets stored. Studies have shown that people of African ethnicity have less visceral fat than others (Sun et al., 2021).

Let us take Mr. A as an example. A middle-aged man who loves his nightly beer routine coupled with chips for a snack may seem harmless at first glance, but slowly, he starts noticing changes—difficulty climbing stairs or feeling tired frequently despite enough rest. A visit to his doctor reveals increased blood glucose levels and high cholesterol—all red flags indicative of excess belly fat.

A waist size of more than 35 inches (89 centimetres) in women and 40 inches (104 centimetres) in men is a sign of visceral obesity and a greater risk of health problems. Age and gender also affect the accumulation of visceral belly fat (*Belly Fat in Women*, 2023). The most common measures to determine if an individual is carrying excess visceral fat include the circumference of the waist, waist-to-hip ratio, and waist-to-hip ratio adjusted for body mass index (BMI) (Sun et al., 2021). Thus, a visually lean person can also carry dangerous quantities of fat in the abdominal region. Studies show visceral fat increases with age (*Belly Fat in Women*, 2023). CT scans and full-body MRIs provide a more accurate measure of visceral fat, but they are expensive and not easily accessible.

Now, let us venture deeper into why this notorious type of fat matters so much.

Studies show that individuals with excess belly fat have higher chances of developing insulin resistance, leading to type 2 diabetes. These fats release chemicals called cytokines that increase risk factors associated with heart disease by raising blood pressure levels and lowering good cholesterol (HDL). (*Abdominal Fat*, 2019).

A study published by the American Journal of Clinical Nutrition in 2023, found that a low-carbohydrate diet has a greater effect on getting rid of visceral fat when compared to a low-fat diet (Oliveira et al., 2023). In another study, just twelve weeks of regular practice of basic yoga among women was found to be directly correlated to reduced abdominal fat, waist-to-hip ratio, and total body fat, along with a substantial increase in muscle mass and improved overall mental well-being (Cramer et al., 2016).

Key Takeaways

- Belly fat is not just about appearance; it's a potential ticking time bomb for various health conditions, such as diabetes and cardiovascular disease.

- High calorific intake coupled with a lack of physical activity are responsible for stubborn belly fat.

- Genetics and age play a role in belly fat.

- Regular physical activity combined with a low-carbohydrate diet has the potential to decrease visceral fat.

Chapter 4:

The Science Behind Belly Fat—Exploring the Biological Factors

Belly fat is no longer viewed merely as an aesthetic nuisance, a cosmetic flaw that prevents our jeans from fitting properly. In recent years, science has unveiled the darker side of belly fat. It is not just about appearances anymore; biological factors are at play. Picture your body as an apple. The skin represents subcutaneous fat—it is right under the skin, harmless yet stubborn. Visceral fat is like the core of the apple—it surrounds vital organs such as the liver, intestines, and pancreas. Visceral fat behaves differently than its benign cousin, subcutaneous fat. Think of visceral fat as a sleeping dragon inside you, silently wreaking havoc on your health while you are unaware.

Let us step into why this happens:

Firstly, unlike passive subcutaneous fat, visceral fat is metabolically active and affects how our hormones function. Imagine it like a chemical factory incessantly pumping out harmful substances into your bloodstream—inflammatory compounds and hormones that can adversely affect your body's function. Secondly, these chemicals lead to insulin resistance over time—a condition where our cells stop responding to insulin hormones correctly, leading to higher blood sugar levels; this situation increases chances of type 2 diabetes. Additionally, these fatty acids move through the liver, affecting its function, leading to cholesterol problems, and triggering inflammation that could cause heart disease (Item & Konrad, 2012).

Now that we have uncovered what belly fat does, let us look at what we can do to ward off this sneaky enemy.

The solution comes from lifestyle changes. Regular exercise helps burn these fats, while a balanced diet prevents further accumulation. Avoiding processed foods, sugars, and unhealthy fats while increasing your intake of whole grains, lean proteins, fruits, and vegetables can go a long way towards keeping belly fat at bay. Regarding exercise, high-intensity interval training (HIIT) has shown promising results in reducing visceral fat, specifically. If belly fat becomes persistent despite efforts, it could signify an underlying hormonal imbalance or metabolic issues for which professional medical advice should be sought. Here is an advanced tip: Incorporating stress-reducing practices like yoga or meditation can help, as stress triggers the cortisol hormone, leading to more visceral fat storage.

Key Takeaways

- Belly fat is not innocuous; it is metabolically active, secreting harmful substances.

- This activity leads to insulin resistance, liver problems, and heart diseases.

- The culprit behind its accumulation is excess calorie intake because of our body's survival mechanism.

- Combat strategies include regular exercise (especially HIIT), a balanced diet, avoiding stress, and seeking professional help if necessary.

Remember, as the old saying goes, "Prevention is better than cure." Understanding the science behind belly fat can empower us to live healthier lives.

Chapter 5:
The Role of Genetics in Accumulating Belly Fat

Have you ever wondered why some people seem to gain weight easily, particularly around the belly area, even when they eat a balanced diet and exercise regularly? Or do you know someone who eats junk food all day but never seems to gain an inch on their waistline? If so, you are not alone. Many people wonder about these apparent inconsistencies. Well, the answer comes from our genes. Genetics plays a significant role in determining where we store fat in our bodies. It is like our bodies have pre-determined storage units for excess calories, and unfortunately for some of us, that unit is located right around the midsection. To understand this further, let us dive into the world of genetics.

Our DNA is like a blueprint that guides how we grow and develop throughout our lives. Just as it determines your hair colour or eye colour, it also influences your body shape and size, including where your body stores fat. Some people are genetically predisposed to carry excess weight in their bellies rather than elsewhere on their bodies. Scientific studies have identified certain genes associated with obesity and belly fat. For instance, one such gene called "FTO" has been nicknamed the "fatso" gene because variations of this gene have been linked to higher levels of obesity. (Lan et al., 2020). Patterns of fat deposits vary between different ethnicities, and thus, individuals of different ancestries are prone to various obesity-linked metabolic syndromes. For example, with increasing BMI, the chances of hypertension and diabetes are greater in Asians compared to non-Hispanic whites, blacks, and Hispanics. Thus, genetic ancestry influences visceral fat and is capable of increasing the risk of metabolic ailments linked to high levels of obesity (Sun et al., 2021).

However, here is an inspirational quote by motivational speaker Jim Rohn: "Your life does not get better by chance; it gets better by change." This means that while we cannot change our genetics (at least not yet), we can change other factors within our control, such as diet and physical activity, which significantly affect how much belly fat we accumulate. So, if you have been cursed with the 'belly fat' genes, do not lose hope just yet. You might need to work harder than others, but you can still achieve a leaner midsection. It is all about finding what works for your body and sticking to it. Remember that even if the problem is severe (e.g., if you are genetically predisposed to obesity), solutions are always available. In such cases, seeking professional advice from dieticians or doctors may be necessary. Incorrect advice often given in this context is that people with 'bad' genes for belly fat should just give up because they're fighting a losing battle. This is certainly not true. Everyone can improve their health with the right guidance and determination.

So, why do we accumulate belly fat? The answer lies partly in our genes but also significantly in our lifestyle choices. Understanding this will help us find effective ways to combat belly fat and maintain a healthier life.

Key Takeaways

- Our genes strongly influence where we store fat in our bodies.
- Regardless of genetic differences, a proper diet and physical activity can reduce belly fat.
- Lifestyle choices trump bad genes when it comes to fat loss.

Chapter 6:
Why Is Losing Belly Fat So Hard? Unravelling the Mystery

Life often presents us with challenges that seem to have no easy solutions. One such challenge is belly fat, a stubborn foe that resists our best efforts to banish it. You have probably asked yourself numerous times: *Why is losing belly fat so hard?* Today, we are going to unravel this mystery.

As discussed earlier, a burgeoning waist circumference is due to two different types of fat: subcutaneous (under the skin) and visceral (around your internal organs). The latter is particularly concerning as it releases inflammatory substances and hormones that can lead to serious diseases like type 2 diabetes and heart disease. Belly fat releases chemicals called cytokines, which increase the risk of heart disease. Over time, I have noticed some common threads among those who struggle with belly fat. These include unhealthy diets high in processed foods and sugars, a lack of physical activity, stress-induced eating patterns, poor sleep quality, and certain genetic factors. This does not mean you are doomed if these factors are present in your life; they simply highlight areas where changes can be beneficial.

The science behind why losing belly fat seems disproportionately difficult compared to other body fats comes from the nature of the cells themselves. Visceral fat is metabolically more active than other fats. Metabolically active means it responds quickly when you start exercising or altering your diet but, unfortunately, re-accumulates equally fast when old habits creep back in. To illustrate this point further, let me share a study published in 2013. The participants' brain activity was monitored using functional magnetic resonance imaging (fMRI) while facing stressful conditions (Jastreboff et al., 2013). The findings revealed an increase in activity within regions involved in craving and reward whenever the participants felt stressed. This suggests that stress can trigger food cravings, which in turn lead to belly fat accumulation. Since varied factors impact abdominal fat, losing it for good also has to be a steady and concentrated effort.

Martha Beck said, "Every day brings new choices," and this reminds us of our power over belly fat. It may be tough to lose, but it is not impossible. Understanding how belly fat works is the first step towards making informed decisions about diet, exercise, and lifestyle changes.

Now, let us talk about some solutions to tackle this issue. To win the battle against belly fat, you need an action plan that includes a balanced diet, regular physical exercise, and stress management techniques. It's also very important to get adequate sleep every day since a lack of sleep affects hormones that trigger hunger and satiation.

Now, onto actionable steps.

Firstly, commit yourself fully to achieving your goal by setting realistic targets, like losing one pound per week, rather than aiming for drastic overnight changes, which are often unsustainable. Maintain a food diary, noting down everything you eat or drink. This helps identify unhealthy patterns like late-night snacking or excessive sugary drink intake.

Next, stay physically active in your day-to-day life. You do not need to join a gym or run marathons; even simple activities like brisk walking or gardening can make a significant difference.

Lastly, prioritise self-care by ensuring you get enough sleep every night and practicing stress management techniques such as meditation or yoga.

Always keep in mind that it is not about one end goal but consistent progress; every small positive change brings you one step closer to your goal. And most importantly, be patient with yourself—losing belly fat is a journey, not a sprint.

Key Takeaways

- Stress triggers food cravings, leading to belly fat accumulation; hence, managing stress is vital to losing belly fat.

- Lack of sleep influences your hunger hormones, contributing to weight gain.

- Obesity is a global epidemic affecting millions worldwide.

- Small positive changes are key to losing belly fat.

Chapter 7:

Obesity Epidemic—A Global Health Crisis

Here are some alarming statistics: According to WHO data, in 2016, close to 2 billion adults were overweight, with over 650 million of them being obese worldwide (*Obesity and Overweight*, 2024). Such numbers highlight the scale of our battle against obesity.

As you pick up this book, you have commenced on a path to understanding belly fat—from what it is to why we gain it and, more importantly, why it is often stubborn to lose. Today, we explore further an alarming aspect of belly fat: its contribution to the global obesity epidemic. Here is a sea of people. Now, picture half that crowd being overweight or obese. This is not an exaggeration but a sad reality, as World Health Organization statistics reveal that almost half the world's population is battling with weight issues (*Obesity and Overweight*, 2024). The World Health Organization (WHO) uses the standardised Body Mass Index (BMI) measure to define obesity and overweight. BMI is calculated as body weight in kilogrammes over height in metres squared. Normal ranges lie between 18.5 and 24.9 (Hurt, 2010). Obesity is defined as 30kg per metre squared. The economic impact of Overweight and Obesity (OAO) was estimated to be 2.19% of gross domestic product (GDP). At current rates, it is supposed to increase to 3.29% of GDP by 2016 (Okunogbe, 2022). Deaths from cardiovascular disease linked to obesity have risen from 2.2 per 100,000 persons to 6.6 per 100,000 persons in the last 2 decades (*Obesity-related cardiovascular disease*, 2023). The economic costs include direct and indirect medical expenses, including in-patient and outpatient costs, travel for hospital visits, carer costs, and employer costs in the form of absenteeism. At the start of this century, the problem of obesity was more prevalent in developed countries; however, today, it is a global phenomenon.

But before we dive headfirst into this vast ocean of information, let me share some wisdom from Thomas Edison: "The doctor of the future will give no medication but will interest his patients in the care of the human frame and diet and cause and prevention of diseases." It is as apt today as when he said it over 100 years ago.

Now, back to our seascape metaphor for understanding obesity. Picture each person as an island fighting against rising tides (increasing body weight) due mostly to unhealthy eating habits and sedentary lifestyles. What happens when these islands get submerged? They disappear, right? In reality, though, they don't vanish without a trace; instead, they leave behind telltale signs like heart disease, diabetes type II, or even certain types of cancer associated with excessive abdominal fat—much like sunken ships leaving wreckage scattered across the ocean floor.

So, how do we deal with this burgeoning issue? The solution lies somewhere between better understanding our bodies, particularly how belly fat accumulates, and the importance of making healthier lifestyle choices.

Let us start with our enemy: the processed food industry, which often lures us into consuming unhealthy foods under the guise of convenience or taste. These foods are high in sugar and unhealthy fats that contribute to weight gain, particularly around your midsection. It may sound like a Sisyphean task to combat this obesity epidemic, but remember, every journey begins with a single step. Start by replacing processed foods with whole grains, lean proteins, and plenty of fruits and vegetables. When it comes to being active, think of it as an essential daily chore, like brushing your teeth. Even simple activities like walking more or taking stairs instead of elevators can help you burn calories and lose belly fat.

Key Takeaways

- Belly fat contributes significantly to global obesity.
- Unhealthy eating habits and a sedentary lifestyle are the primary culprits.
- The processed food industry is an enemy disguised as convenience.
- Switching to healthier food options and staying active can help combat obesity.

Part II:

Implication of Excessive Belly Fat

Chapter 8:
Diseases Indicated by an Increased Waistline

The human body is a complex machine, a marvel of biological engineering. Even so, it is not immune to misfires and malfunctions. One such malfunction we often see today is fat accumulation around the waistline. Picture your waistline as the "check engine" light in your car. When that light comes on, you know something needs attention under the hood. Similarly, an expanding waistline can indicate something is amiss with your internal machinery.

One potential problem linked to belly fat is heart disease. The American Heart Association has found that people with excess belly fat are at a higher risk of heart disease and stroke than those without it (*More Belly Weight*, 2021). Another study conducted in the United Kingdom involving 500,000 people (aged 40 to 69) found that women who carried more weight around their midsection had a 10% to 20% greater risk of heart attack than women who were just heavier overall (measured by body mass index, or BMI) (Bilodeau, 2018). This study directly links abdominal (visceral) obesity to an increased risk of heart disease. An overall measure of obesity, like BMI, was not found to be a driver of an increased risk of heart disease. It is like driving with faulty brakes; you are bound to crash sooner or later.

Another disease associated with excessive belly fat is type 2 diabetes. In fact, research shows that over 80% of people diagnosed with this condition are overweight or obese. Type 2 diabetes is a condition in which cells become resistant to insulin's signal to move glucose from the blood to the cells to turn it into energy. Excess weight has been found to contribute to it since fat cells affect how the body uses glucose and produces insulin. A lack of physical activity can increase the risk of type 2 diabetes (LeWine, 2012). Though medication can keep type 2 diabetes under control, exercise and normal body weight are often all that is required to combat it. Picture sugar coursing through your veins like sandpaper, slowly wearing down your body's ability to produce insulin effectively.

Furthermore, studies have also linked belly fat to certain types of cancer, such as breast cancer and colon cancer, two heavyweight contenders in the world's most lethal disease arena. Excess visceral fat creates a low-oxygen environment, which creates chronic inflammation. Chronic inflammation increases the chances of tumour formation. Obesity has also been linked to higher levels of oestrogen, which is also linked to various types of cancer in women (Underferth, 2017).

Now that we have painted quite the grim picture, let us lighten up the mood by reminding ourselves that knowledge is power. By knowing these risks associated with increased abdominal obesity, we are better equipped to take action against them. This understanding should serve as motivation rather than intimidation. Remember what Michael Pollan, author of the books that deal with the socio-cultural impact of food, once said: "Eat food. Not too much. Mostly plants." To combat belly fat and the diseases it can lead to, we need to make wiser choices about our nutrition and activity levels. So, if your waistline is expanding and you are concerned about what that could mean for your health, take action. Start by consulting a healthcare provider who can assess your risk factors and guide you through the necessary steps towards a healthier lifestyle.

Do not be disheartened if the problem seems overwhelming or the risk is already severe. It is never too late to turn things around. Consider working with professionals like dieticians or fitness trainers who provide customised plans based on your body type, lifestyle, and preferences.

Key Takeaways

- Excessive abdominal fat is associated with an increased risk of heart disease.

- Overweight or obese individuals are more likely to develop type 2 diabetes.

- Certain types of cancer have been linked to excessive belly fat.

- Knowledge about the problem at hand enables us to make educated decisions regarding our health.

- Consultation with healthcare providers is essential for proper assessment and guidance.

Remember this chapter as not just an enumeration of potential risks but rather as an empowerment tool in your fight against belly fat. The battle may seem daunting now, but remember that every journey begins with a single step, so let us get stepping.

Chapter 9:

The Metabolic Menace

Health is not valued till sickness comes.

-Thomas Fuller

Have you ever wondered why your belly is often the first place to store fat and the last to lose it? As discussed in previous chapters, this is not just an aesthetically unpleasant problem. There is a hidden villain at work here, and its name is metabolic syndrome. Metabolic syndrome is a serious condition that needs immediate attention. It is a host of conditions that put us at greater risk of conditions like coronary illnesses, diabetes, hypertension, and kidney disorders (Lopes, 2016). Excessive belly fat is not just physical appearance; it is an indication that something more sinister might be brewing underneath.

But don't worry. This chapter will help you understand what metabolic syndrome means, how it relates to belly fat, and how you can fight back.

The Invisible Threat

Imagine your body to be a city. Each organ represents a different neighbourhood or district. Imagine if one district started expanding uncontrollably, causing chaos in traffic flow and overburdening resources. That is precisely what happens when we have too much belly fat; it disrupts our internal city's harmony. In scientific terms, having excessive abdominal obesity leads to insulin resistance; very simply put, this means that the pancreas produces insulin—a hormone that regulates how much sugar is absorbed by cells—but cells resist its action, leading to higher levels of sugar in the blood, essentially paving the way for diabetes and heart diseases. Free fatty acids in the bloodstream can also lead to inflammation, which creates a waxy plaque-like substance in the blood vessels, increasing blood pressure and leading to various other diseases of the blood vessels (*Metabolic Syndrome*, 2022).

Unravelling the Solution

Now that we know about metabolic syndrome, let's talk about tackling this menace head-on. First things first, get moving. Regular physical activity helps lower insulin resistance—aim for at least 30 minutes of moderate-intensity exercise every day. Secondly, eat healthily. Opt for a diet rich in fruits, vegetables, lean proteins, and whole grains. Keep processed sugars to a minimum. But remember to consume these within your daily calorie needs. If the problem is extra severe, consider seeking professional help. A nutritionist or a personal trainer can provide you with tailored advice and guidance that suits your body type and lifestyle. Also, avoid falling into the trap of quick-fix solutions like fad diets or extreme workout regimes that promise rapid weight loss. These methods often lead to muscle loss instead of fat loss and are not sustainable in the long run.

Excessive belly fat is not just an eyesore; it is a potential health hazard leading to metabolic syndrome. The remedy to this is not short-term fixes but everyday choices like being physically active and adopting a healthy diet. Remember, health truly is wealth. Let's pledge today to take small yet steady steps towards healthier living because every little bit counts when it comes to maintaining our internal harmony.

Key Takeaways

- Excessive belly fat leads to insulin resistance, contributing to metabolic syndrome.
- Metabolic syndrome requires immediate attention.
- Regular physical activity helps regulate hormones like insulin.
- A balanced diet within your daily calorie needs assists in managing belly fat.
- Avoid quick-fix solutions that are not sustainable in the long run.

Chapter 10:
How Belly Fat Affects Your Heart, Liver, and Other Organs

Welcome to the heart of our discussion on belly fat. You might be wondering why we are delving into the details of how excess weight around your midsection affects your internal organs. Well, it is because belly fat has far-reaching implications for your overall health. Visceral fat gives us real cause for concern. That is because this type of fat is biochemically active.

Now, let us take a deep dive into what happens when we have excessive amounts of this stubborn flab, hugging our vital organs. When you carry excess weight around your abdomen, it puts unnecessary pressure on your heart, making it work harder to pump blood throughout your body. This extra strain can lead to elevated levels of blood pressure and other cardiovascular problems—which is the leading cause of death worldwide. Then, there is the connection between belly fat and liver health. When too much visceral fat builds up in your abdomen, some inevitably spill over into the liver, causing fatty liver disease—a condition where excess fats build up inside cells in this vital organ, impairing its function over time. The effects do not stop at cardiovascular health or even liver damage, though; research has shown links between increased waist circumference (a measure used by doctors as a proxy for abdominal obesity) and an array of conditions, including certain types of cancer.

The evidence is difficult to ignore. A study published by the Harvard Medical School found that for a 2-inch increase in waist circumference, cardiovascular disease risk increased by 10% in women, even after adjusting for body mass index (BMI) (*Taking Aim*, 2024). This shows just how significant an indicator of belly fat is for overall health risks.

Let's look at some real-life examples. Take Jim, a 45-year-old man with a big belly who seemed healthy otherwise. He was shocked when his doctor told him he was at high risk for heart disease because of his abdominal obesity. Or consider Anna, a middle-aged woman who struggled with fat loss and eventually developed type-2 diabetes—all because of her excess visceral fat.

Now that we've established the problem, let us explore potential solutions.

One approach is regular exercise—particularly activities that get your heart rate up, like brisk walking or cycling. When combined with a healthy diet full of fruits, vegetables, unprocessed grains, and lean proteins, this can help reduce body fat in general, including persistent abdominal fat. White adipose tissues (WAT), which serve as energy reserves in the body, make up visceral fat. Brown adipose tissue (BAT), on the other hand, actively burns fat to keep the body insulated. Exposure to cold weather, good nutrition, and a healthy lifestyle can help convert white fat cells into brown cells, thereby stimulating energy expenditure (Thyagarajan & Foster, 2017).

Case studies have repeatedly proven this strategy effective. For example, one study published in Obesity Reviews found that adults who combined aerobic exercise with resistance training lost significantly more visceral fat than those who did either alone (Brown et al., 2009).

A Harvard Medical School study states that having a waist size over 40 inches for men or 35 inches for women puts you at risk for heart disease even if your BMI falls within the "normal" range (*Waist Size Matters*, 2012).

Here are some interesting points to note:

- Not all calories are created equal; eating certain foods like omega 3 fatty acids and apple cider vinegar could stimulate 'beiging', the process that turns white (bad) fat into brown (good) fat (Blessing et al., 2012).

- Stress plays a role in weight gain; high levels of cortisol (the stress hormone) have been linked to increased abdominal obesity (*The Stress-Diet Connection*, 2020).

- Genetics matter too; genes affect where you store fat, and some people are genetically predisposed to carry excess weight around their middle (Blessing et al., 2012).

Now, let us talk about specific steps you can take:

1. Start moving: Aim to include 30 minutes of moderate-to-high-intensity physical activity 3-4 days a week.

2. Refine your diet: Reduce the intake of processed foods high in added sugars and unhealthy fats. Opt for unprocessed food items like whole grains, fruits, vegetables, and lean proteins.

3. Get enough sleep. Studies suggest that a lack of sleep may increase the risk of obesity.

4. Manage stress: try relaxation techniques like yoga or meditation to keep cortisol levels in check.

5. Regular check-ups: regularly monitor your waist circumference and other vital health indicators.

Remember, it's not about perfection but progression. So, start small, make consistent efforts each day, and gradually build healthier habits that will help you lose belly fat sustainably while improving overall wellness.

Key Takeaways

- Excess visceral or "belly" fat is much more dangerous than subcutaneous fat because of its location near vital organs such as the heart and liver.

- Regular exercise combined with a balanced diet are powerful tools against belly fat.

- Belly fat is influenced by more than just diet and exercise. Stress and genetics come into play too.

- The belly fat problem is widespread across genders and ages.

Chapter 11:
Mental Health Concerns Related to Obesity

In my journey within the realm of health and fitness, I have come across numerous misconceptions about this stubborn adipose tissue that clings to your midsection. Interestingly, while many are aware of its visible implications, few understand the hidden dangers lurking beneath, especially when it comes to mental health.

We have discussed how belly fat contributes significantly to chronic diseases like diabetes and heart problems. But did you ever stop to consider what effect it could have on your brain? Research has found compelling links between obesity and various psychological disorders, including depression, anxiety, and even severe conditions like schizophrenia (Hajek, 2021).

Now, let us get into the meat of this issue.

Belly fat increases inflammation in your body, which can lead to cognitive decline over time. As far as mental health issues are concerned, scientists believe that inflammation might be a significant contributing factor. This is because inflammatory markers are frequently elevated in people suffering from depression or anxiety disorders (Hajek, 2021).

The scientific literature abounds with evidence supporting these claims. For instance, a study published in the American Academy of Neurology in 2019 found that individuals with higher waist-to-hip ratios (indicative of increased belly fat) had lower brain volumes compared to those with less belly fat.

Consider Jane Doe, for example (name changed for privacy). Jane was an energetic woman who loved her job as a marketing executive until she started gaining weight because of hormonal imbalances after childbirth. Despite maintaining an active lifestyle post-pregnancy, Jane noticed an increasing girth around her waistline, which began affecting her self-esteem, eventually leading to periods of depression and anxiety.

Naomi Judd's saying, "Your body hears everything your mind says," reminds us that our physical health directly impacts our mental well-being. The science behind these words is simple: excess belly fat secretes inflammatory substances, causing systemic inflammation, which in turn increases the risk of mental health disorders.

Now, let us take a look at another case study from a report published in the Journal of Clinical Psychiatry. This study found that the occurrence of depression in males over 40 years of age is directly correlated to abdominal obesity (Vogelzangs et al., 2008). These findings show that addressing obesity can potentially reduce certain mental health conditions.

Here are some interesting bullet points to remember:

- Belly fat can induce inflammation throughout our bodies.

- Inflammation is correlated with mental health conditions like depression and anxiety.

- Losing belly fat not only improves your physique but also benefits your brain health.

Consider this statistic: A staggering 40% of adults were overweight in 2016, and close to a third of them were obese. These numbers highlight the severity of the obesity epidemic we are facing today (*World Obesity Day, 2022*).

So, how do you take action? Here are some steps:

1. Start by getting regular exercise; aim for at least half an hour most days.

2. Eat balanced meals loaded with fibre, like fruits, vegetables, and whole grains.

3. Restrict the intake of processed foods high in sugar and unhealthy fats, as they contribute to weight gain.

4. Practice mindfulness eating: eat slowly, savour each bite, listen to hunger cues, and stop when full.

5. If you have been following the above steps and are still struggling with the process, consider seeking professional help from a dietician, a mental health counsellor, or both.

Remember, every step towards a healthier lifestyle is a step closer to improved mental well-being. So, let us start taking those steps today.

Key Takeaways

- The relationship between belly fat and mental health is not merely coincidental but rather causal—one leads to another.

- Belly fat is not just a matter of physical appearance. It plays a pivotal role in determining our physical, mental, and spiritual states.

- Mental wellness is interconnected with physical wellness; losing belly fat could be a stepping stone towards better overall health.

- Obesity is not just an individual problem; it's a global public health issue that needs immediate action.

Part III:
Analysing Triggers for Developing Visceral Fat

Chapter 12:
Sedentary Lifestyle and Its Effects on Body Weight

Our modern lives are filled with conveniences that make movement optional. Easy access to food, remote controls, elevators and escalators, and online shopping have created an environment promoting a sedentary lifestyle. But remember, just because we can choose stillness doesn't mean it is the best choice for our health. Think of your body as a classic car. It needs regular maintenance and fuel to function optimally like any other vehicle. Imagine leaving this car idle in your garage for months or even years without using it. What happens? The battery goes flat; tyres deflate; oil becomes gummy; belts crack and rot from non-use—the car deteriorates faster than if used regularly. Similarly, when we lead sedentary lifestyles—sitting at desks all day, watching TV for hours on end—our bodies begin to break down from lack of use. It is like living life stuck in park gear.

The Science Behind Sedentarism

A study published in Obesity has proven that leading a sedentary lifestyle is one of the key triggers for developing visceral fat, or belly fat. A sedentary lifestyle has been linked to higher mortality rates. People who sit for longer periods tend to have higher levels of belly fat (Whitaker et al., 2017). Another study concluded that every additional hour spent sitting daily was linked with a nearly two per cent increase in the presence of belly fat (Henson et al., 2017). In simple terms, sitting is not just making us larger around the middle—it is also killing us slowly.

This brings us back to Albert Einstein's quote, "Life is like riding a bicycle. To keep your balance, you must keep moving." The human body was designed to move—not sit for extended periods. When we don't move, our bodies begin to store excess calories as fat, particularly around the abdomen.

The less sedentary, the better.

So, what should you do if your lifestyle is extra-sedentary? What if you are chained to a desk job or are unable to engage in regular physical exercise because of health conditions?

Start small. Even minor adjustments can have significant effects over time. Aim to stay active all through the day. Make little changes to your everyday routines, like walking up the stairs instead of taking the elevator, stretching your body in between bouts of sitting, and taking breaks for yourself to take a stroll or go on a short run. Use stairs instead of elevators when possible (Dempsey et al., 2016). Light resistance exercises use large muscle groups almost 20 times as much as sitting and positively impact energy expenditure and glucose uptake. These small changes can help break the inactivity cycle and reduce belly fat accumulation. Bodyweight half-squats, calf raises, gluteal contractions, and knee raises can all be incorporated into your day to keep your body in motion. Studies also found that the increased mortality risk arising from prolonged hours of sitting can be offset by spending a sufficiently high amount of time on moderately intense physical activity (an hour a day). Thus, the negative impact of sedentary time is also found to be higher in individuals who do not engage in moderate to vigorous physical activity (Henson et al., 2017).

However, remember that while movement is beneficial, it is not always about burning calories—it is about maintaining functionality and overall health.

Key Takeaways

> - Leading a sedentary lifestyle contributes significantly to the development of belly fat.
>
> - Sitting for extended periods has detrimental effects on our health.
>
> - Even minor movements or exercises can have significant effects over time.

Chapter 13:
Stress Eating and Emotional Overeating—Unhealthy Coping Mechanisms

They say that laughter is the best medicine, but for many people, it is food. After a long, stressful day at work or when dealing with emotional turmoil, the first instinct is often to reach out for that tub of ice cream or bag of chips. This chapter aims to explore how stress and emotions can trigger overeating and lead to belly fat accumulation.

Stress eating, also known as emotional eating, is consuming large quantities of food—usually 'comfort' or junk foods—in response to feelings instead of hunger. It is like having a hole in your heart that you are trying to fill with food. Interestingly enough, there is a science behind why we do this. When faced with a challenging situation, the body releases adrenaline, which sends us into a fight or flight mode to face the imminent danger. Immediately following, our body produces excess amounts of cortisol, a hormone that increases glucose in our blood to provide increased energy. However, cortisol also increases the urge to reach out for foods high in sugar, salt, and fat. These foods give us a burst of energy and pleasure by increasing "feel-good" hormones like serotonin in our brains (*The Stress-Diet Connection*, 2020).

"Food is not just calories; it is information. It actually contains messages that connect to every cell in the body," says Dr. Mark Hyman. Thus, every bite tells us how to behave. And unfortunately, stress tells us all the wrong things. Consequently, these temporary moments of satisfaction are quickly replaced by guilt about overeating and worries about weight gain, which further fuel the cycle, thus leading to an unhealthy relationship with food. Emotional eating is an unhealthy coping mechanism triggered by stress and negative emotions, leading directly towards weight gain, primarily around the belly area, due to its influence on our hormonal balance.

So, how do we break free from this vicious cycle? Here are some actionable steps:

1. Identify triggers: The first step towards solving any problem is identifying what causes it. Keep a journal detailing what you eat, when you eat it, what triggered your urge to eat, and how you feel after eating.

2. Develop healthy coping mechanisms: Rather than turning to food, engage in activities that can help reduce stress, like yoga, meditation, or going for a walk.

3. Mindful eating: Being mindful of the process of eating means approaching it as an experience to savour. Take note of the effects of food both within and outside of your body. It may include noticing colours, smells, textures, and flavours and how they make you feel.

4. Seek professional help: If emotional eating has become a significant part of your life, consider seeking help from a psychologist or a licensed counsellor specialising in emotional eating.

Remember, changing habits takes time. Be patient with yourself and celebrate small victories along the way.

If things get worse and overeating starts affecting your overall health, severely causing obesity-related complications like diabetes or heart disease, it is best to see a doctor immediately who might suggest more intensive treatments like weight-loss medication or surgery. The enemy here is not food but our relationship with it. It is important to understand that no amount of dieting will work if we do not address the underlying issues triggering unhealthy eating habits.

Key Takeaways

- Stress triggers hormonal imbalances, leading to cravings for unhealthy foods.

- Emotional overeating is often a way to suppress negative feelings.

- Steps towards managing stress eating include identifying possible triggers, practising the art of being fully present while eating, and adopting healthier coping mechanisms.

- If emotional overeating becomes severe, seeking professional help is recommended.

Chapter 14:

Impact of Alcohol, Smoking, and Drug Use on Weight Gain

The attempt to escape from pain, is what creates more pain.

-Gabor Maté

Let us explore further some triggers that contribute largely to developing visceral fat: alcohol, smoking, and drugs. These are prevalent in today's society, and their impact on weight gain is a topic worth exploring.

Alcohol has been a part of human culture for centuries, seen as an elixir for social bonding or a comforting solace at the end of a long day. However, it also bears an infamous reputation for its role in adding those extra pounds around your waistline. This could be attributed to its high-calorie content—seven per gramme—almost equal to fat. Not only this, but alcohol can interfere with the body's natural fat-burning process (Traversy & Chaput, 2018). The intensity of drinking per session is significant for fat accumulation.

Similarly, smoking tobacco cigarettes is often associated with staying in shape because nicotine helps reduce appetite and boost metabolism. But do not be fooled! Research shows that smokers tend to have more abdominal fat compared to non-smokers because of the complex interplay between nicotine and insulin function (Carrasquilla et al., 2024). Lastly, drug use can lead to weight gain by causing changes in physical activity levels or eating patterns while disrupting normal body functions.

A study conducted by The American Journal of Clinical Nutrition found that individuals who consumed more than three drinks daily had 80% higher chances of having excess belly fat than those who drank less often (Sonko et al., 1994). Similarly, research published in PLOS One journal showed that former smokers had larger waist circumferences compared to non-smokers, albeit less than current smokers (Chatkin et al., 2015). A study published in The Journal of Pharmacology and Experimental Therapeutics found that alcohol consumption decreased whole-body lipid oxidation (a measure of how much fat your body is burning) by more than 70% (Lockett, 2023). Another study indicated that nicotine impairs glucose homeostasis, leading to abdominal obesity.

For instance, consider John Doe, a healthy young adult who enjoyed his casual beer every evening until he noticed his pants getting tighter over time without any significant change in diet or exercise routine. Or Jane Smith, an ex-smoker, noticed her waistline expanding post-quitting, a phenomenon often referred to as "quit smoking weight gain."

Analysing these triggers reveals that they essentially disrupt our body's balance. Alcohol, with its empty calories and interference in fat burning, smoking through altered insulin function, and drugs by changing physical activity or eating patterns all lead to that unwanted belly fat.

- Moderate drinking can result in significant calorie intake.
- Smoking could lead to insulin resistance, promoting visceral fat.
- Drug use may alter physical activity or diet patterns, contributing to weight gain.

Several studies reveal startling facts about this issue. One such study suggests that globally, over two billion people consume alcohol, with nearly 63% indulging excessively (Traversy & Chaput, 2018). This shows why addressing this trigger is crucial when tackling belly fat issues worldwide.

For an actionable plan:

1. Limit alcohol: Stick to moderate drinking, defined as up to 10 grammes and 20 grammes of alcohol per day for women and men, respectively.

2. Quit smoking: Seek professional help if struggling with quitting; consider alternatives like nicotine patches or gums.

3. Drug-free lifestyle: Maintain a healthy lifestyle free from illicit drug use; seek help immediately if battling addiction.

4. A regular exercise routine and a balanced diet are the cornerstones of managing your weight effectively.

5. Consider professional help, therapy, and meditation to reduce stress and learn healthy coping mechanisms instead of turning to addictive behaviour patterns.

Understanding these triggers and their impact on our body can help us make better decisions to manage our belly fat. Remember, every small step counts when it comes to your health. So, take that first step today and start the effort you put in towards a healthier you.

Key Takeaways

- Alcohol, smoking, and drugs contribute significantly to belly fat accumulation through various mechanisms, like high caloric intake from alcohol or altered insulin functioning because of smoking.

- These triggers disrupt normal bodily functions, leading to an increased accumulation of visceral fat.

- Understanding these factors can help in devising effective strategies for managing belly fat.

- The global prevalence of these triggers necessitates their inclusion while addressing weight management strategies on a larger scale.

Chapter 15:
Sleep Deprivation and Its Correlation With Obesity

Sleep deprivation is a silent assassin, silently taking a toll on our health. It is not just about feeling grumpy or under-caffeinated; sleep deficiency can result in packing on those pounds, especially around the midsection. In fact, there is a fascinating correlation between sleep deprivation and obesity that often goes unnoticed. In this chapter, we are going to lift the veil on this underappreciated relationship.

Picture your body as an intricate machine. When you deprive it of sleep—it is much-needed downtime for repair and restoration—things start to fall out of balance. When you are chronically sleep-deprived, two key hormones regulating hunger—leptin and ghrelin—get thrown out of whack. Leptin indicates satiation, while ghrelin gives signals to the body as to when to eat. Lack of sleep decreases leptin levels while increasing ghrelin—a double whammy leading to an increased appetite (van Egmond et al., 2022). To put it simply, imagine these hormones as two friends in a car on a long road trip where Leptin is driving. As long as both are well rested (Leptin is alert at the wheel), they keep each other in check (Ghrelin does not ask for unnecessary pit stops for snacks). But when they are tired (sleep-deprived), Ghrelin takes over the steering wheel, demanding more food breaks than necessary.

A study from the University of Chicago found that people who were sleep-deprived consumed almost 300 extra calories per day compared to those who got adequate rest. Sleep-deprived individuals were found to reach out for snacks almost 33% in excess of the calories needed for the extra wakeful hours. This was noticed in spite of the participants having consumed up to 90% of the total calorie requirement two hours prior (Hanlon, 2016). That is like eating an additional cheeseburger every day.

But it gets worse. Sleep deprivation also affects insulin resistance—your cells' ability to respond properly to insulin—leading to higher blood sugar levels and creating a vicious cycle of weight gain. If this does not convince you to prioritise sleep, remember the wise words of Arianna Huffington: "Sleep your way to the top." While she meant it in terms of professional success, it rings true for achieving weight-loss goals too. Lipids synthesised by the sleep-deprived body activate the same receptors that are activated by marijuana.

Now that we have uncovered this hidden enemy, what should you do if you are caught in this destructive cycle?

- Prioritise Sleep: Ensure you wind down and relax before bedtime. This may include having a calming bedtime routine, including journaling, skin care, reading, and any other soothing activities you enjoy. Deep sleep usually takes place in cycles of 90 minutes. Try not to set an alarm in between a 90-minute cycle. Try to aim for a minimum of five 90-minute cycles of undisturbed sleep.

- Time your last meal of the day at least two hours before sleeping. This way, the body gets enough time to digest the meal before unwinding for rest.

- Limit Screen Time Before Bed: It is advisable to keep gadgets aside for at least an hour before retiring to bed. The blue light emitted by screens can imitate sunlight and disrupt your sleep by interrupting the production of melatonin, the sleep hormone.

- Use white noise and a sleeping eye mask for a night of undisturbed sleep. Consider using calming essential oils like lavender and avoiding any stimulants for a relaxed night of sleep.

- Stay Active: Regular physical activity helps regulate your body's circadian rhythm, promoting better sleep. Aim to sleep at the same time every night. This creates a routine that is easier to stick to.

- Seek professional help. If you are still struggling with sleep issues, talk to a healthcare provider.

There is no denying that getting adequate shuteye plays a critical role in maintaining optimal health and managing our waistlines. So, let us commit today not just to diet and exercise but also to prioritising good-quality rest every night as part of our holistic approach towards fighting the battle against belly fat.

Key Takeaways

- Chronic sleep deprivation can lead to weight gain, especially belly fat.

- Lack of enough rest disrupts the balance between the hunger-regulating hormones leptin and ghrelin.

- Inadequate sleep also increases insulin resistance, which further contributes to weight gain.

- Adopting healthy sleeping habits is crucial to combating obesity.

Part IV:

Dietary Considerations for

Reducing Abdominal Bulge

Chapter 16:
Food Habits That Lead to Excess Pounds

What we eat makes a world of difference in our bodies, especially when it comes to belly fat. It is like a balloon that fills up with every bite of the wrong food. Imagine feeding your body the fuel it needs rather than burdening it with excess baggage. Our diet is often the biggest culprit behind bulging bellies. Our modern lifestyle has led us down a path of convenience, where fast food and processed snacks reign supreme. These foods are loaded with sugar, unhealthy fats, and empty calories, which contribute significantly to abdominal weight gain.

So, let us step into understanding these harmful eating habits that lead to excess pounds in your abdomen area:

1. Consuming Too Much Sugar: It's the sweet poison that sneaks into our diet unnoticed through soft drinks, candies, pastries, and even some fruits. Our body converts this sugar into fat around our middle section.

2. Eating Refined Grains: White bread, pasta, or rice might taste great, but they're stripped of their fibre content, making them quickly digest sugars, which eventually turn into belly fat.

3. Binge Eating: Large meals put pressure on your digestive system, leading to bloating and an enlarged stomach over time.

4. Lack of Protein: Carbohydrates are a quick source of energy. However, proteins take longer to digest and release energy. The body expends calories to process proteins, which helps aid in weight loss.

5. Late-Night Snacking: Eating late at night keeps your metabolism active, which causes indigestion and increases your waistline over time.

But what if you are already stuck in this vicious cycle of unhealthy eating habits and an expanding belly? By shifting our focus from 'what not to eat' towards 'what to eat', we can start making healthier choices. Fear not; it is never too late to make a change. Here are some simple steps you can start with:

1. Swap the sugars: Replace your sugar-loaded drinks with water or green tea, which aid in detoxification and weight loss.

2. Choose whole grains: Opt for whole-grain bread and brown rice, which take longer to digest and keep you full for longer.

3. Including foods rich in soluble fibres like oats, fruits, and vegetables can keep you satiated for longer.

4. Small portions: Try having smaller meals at regular intervals instead of two or three large meals.

5. Protein power: Incorporate lean proteins like chicken, fish, tofu, or lentils into your diet.

6. Time your meals: Stop consuming food at least two to three hours before retiring to sleep, allowing efficient assimilation of the ingested food.

7. Stay hydrated. It is quite common for thirst to be confused with hunger. Thus, staying hydrated can help eliminate over-eating based on false hunger cues.

Remember that these changes will not happen overnight, but persistence is key. As Charles Duhigg said, "Change might not be fast, and it is not always easy. But with time and effort, almost any habit can be reshaped." Start by taking small steps: replace your soda with water or opt for stairs instead of elevators; incorporate resistance training exercises into your workout regime; keep track of what you eat; and ensure adequate sleep, as a lack of rest increases cravings for high-calorie foods. Remember, Rome wasn't built overnight. Slow and steady wins the race.

Key Takeaways

- Belly fat accumulation is largely linked to dietary choices.

- Unhealthy food habits include high sugar intake, consuming refined grains, binge eating, and late-night snacking.

- Make healthier swaps, such as choosing water over sugary drinks and opting for whole grains over refined ones.

- Incorporate more proteins into your diet while timing your meals right to prevent midnight snacking.

Remember that every bite you take matters, so let us choose wisely.

Chapter 17:

Superfood Compounds That Fight Against Obesity; Spotlight on Anthocyanin

Before we explore the depths of this chapter, let us consider a quote by Hippocrates, the father of medicine: "Let food be thy medicine, and medicine be thy food." It is a simple yet profound statement that reminds us to think about what we consume. While our primary aim in eating may be to satiate hunger, it is also an opportunity for us to nourish our bodies and support good health.

In previous chapters, we have learned about belly fat—why it is so stubborn, how it can lead to diseases like diabetes and heart conditions, and strategies for losing it effectively. But now, let's turn our attention towards superfoods—not the ones hyped up by media outlets or influencers but backed by science as useful in fighting obesity. In our tireless quest to shed stubborn belly fat, we often overlook the potent possibilities offered by Mother Nature. Superfoods, nutrient-rich foods considered beneficial for health and well-being, come packed with compounds that can wage a formidable war against obesity.

Did you know that certain types of fat can actually help us lose weight? It sounds counter-intuitive but bear with me. Let us take omega-3 fatty acids found in seeds like flax, hemp, and chia and fatty freshwater fish like salmon. These essential fats contribute to feelings of fullness, controlling overeating while also enhancing metabolic functions (Couet et al., 1997).

Now, let us explore the world of superfoods and their belly-busting potential further.

Quinoa, for instance, is a treasure trove of proteins—an essential nutrient renowned for its satiety-inducing properties and metabolic boost. Similarly, blueberries offer high fibre content and host anthocyanins believed to prevent obesity and diabetes. Cast your memory back to your childhood days when spinach was simply a green, leafy nightmare on your plate. Well, Popeye had it right all along. Spinach possesses thylakoids that can slow down fat digestion, prompting hormones that make us feel fuller (Rebello, 2015). Take these superfoods as examples rather than exceptions, proving the rule—food is not always the enemy; it can be part of the solution, too.

Analysing our dietary habits reveals one crucial factor contributing significantly to abdominal bulge: processed foods high in sugars and unhealthy fats, leading inevitably towards weight gain. Replacing these calorific catastrophes with nutrient-dense superfoods could pave a path towards healthier body composition. Consider real-life examples of people who have made this switch. Sarah, a 35-year-old woman, managed to shed over 30 pounds simply by incorporating superfoods into her diet and eliminating processed foods. Similarly, many studies, like the one published in *North American Journal of Medical Sciences*, confirm the potent anti-obesity effects of natural food compounds (Li et al., 2011).

To leverage these benefits:

- Incorporate a variety of superfoods into your daily diet; diversity confirms nutrient sufficiency.

- Limit intake of processed foods; they contain large quantities of sugars and saturated fats.

- Hydrate adequately; water aids digestion and promotes feelings of fullness.

- Along with dietary changes, regular physical activities should be added for better results.

Here is some food for thought:

- Green tea contains catechins that boost metabolism and aid fat burning.

- Greek yoghurt is high in protein, promoting satiety and lean muscle development.

- Avocados are rich in monounsaturated fats, reducing abdominal fat storage.

In all my experience dealing with nutritional matters, I have come to realise one undeniable fact: no single solution fits all when it comes to fat loss, but leveraging the power presented by nature through superfoods certainly gives us an edge against obesity. So, gear up, munch on these nutritional powerhouses, and bid adieu to that stubborn belly fat.

Power of Anthocyanin

Anthocyanins are compounds that naturally occur in many fruits and vegetables and give them their vibrant red, purple, and blue hues. Think blueberries, grapes, black rice, or eggplant—you are essentially seeing anthocyanins at work. But these compounds are not just there for aesthetic purposes; they keep the cells of the body healthy by protecting them from free radicals. It has antioxidative and anti-inflammatory attributes that help protect your cells from oxidative damage. And when it comes to obesity? They are practically superheroes.

Picture this: You are in a vibrant market, and your eyes are drawn to the deep reds, purples, and blues of a fruit stall. These colours are not just pleasing to look at; they represent a powerful group of compounds called anthocyanins found in superfoods. They may be key to reducing your belly fat. Anthocyanins belong to the bioactive family known as flavonoids; plant pigments responsible for splashing our fruits with beautiful hues. But these natural dyes do more than beautify our plates; research shows they can also help reduce obesity by targeting abdominal fat.

Now let us delve into why we need anthocyanins in our battle against belly fat. Abdominal obesity is not just an aesthetic concern; it is linked with many diseases like diabetes and heart disease. And here is something you already know from previous chapters: Belly fat is notoriously stubborn because it consists mainly of adipose tissue designed for long-term energy storage. Anthocyanins are potent antioxidants that have been extensively studied for their health benefits, including their anti-inflammatory properties and their potential role in weight management. Evidence supporting these claims is abundant. In one study published in The Journal of Nutritional Biochemistry, rats fed high-fat diets supplemented with blackberry extract (rich in anthocyanins) showed reduced weight gain compared to those without the supplement (Trinei et al., 2022).

Take Mary, for instance. A mother of two who struggled with post-pregnancy weight gain embarked on a diet rich in berries after reading about the benefits of anthocyanin. Within six months, she noticed significant changes not only in her appearance but also in her overall wellness.

Analysing the role of anthocyanin further, it becomes clear that their potential goes beyond just weight management. They interact with various biological pathways to boost overall health. Consider the research conducted by Tsuda et al. (2003), wherein mice fed an anthocyanin-rich diet showed reduced abdominal fat and triglyceride levels. A study by Mykkänen et al. (2014) linked berry consumption to improved insulin sensitivity.

Interesting fact about anthocyanins:

- It is found in deeply coloured fruits such as blackberries, blueberries, and cherries.

- It is a potent antioxidant.

- It has demonstrated anti-inflammatory properties.

- It plays a potential role in weight management.

Now, let us talk numbers. A review published in *Nutrients* reported that individuals with high flavonoid intake had fewer risks of fatty liver caused by dietary habits, comorbidities associated with obesity, and type 2 diabetes (Sandoval et al., 2020). In addition, Harvard researchers found that increased berry consumption correlated with less weight gain among women over time (Ivey et al., 2017).

Remember, your health is an investment, not an expense.

Scientific research supports the effectiveness of flavonoid-rich foods for weight control. One study shows that people consuming higher amounts of flavonoid-rich foods gained significantly less weight compared to those who consumed less (Bertoia et al., 2016).

Scientific studies have shown that anthocyanins can help with fat loss by enhancing fat burning and reducing fat storage (Tsuda et al., 2003). They can moderate blood sugar levels, thereby curbing overeating because of sudden drops in glucose, and boost your metabolism too (Ivey et al., 2017). Think of your body as a city with bustling traffic. The cars represent the fats circulating in your body, while traffic lights control their movement. In simple terms, anthocyanins act like efficient traffic controllers who make sure fats do not pile up, causing "traffic jams" (think: excess belly fat), but instead guide them towards routes where they'll be used as fuel for your bodily activities. What is more, anthocyanins have been studied for their potential role in reducing risk factors associated with obesity-related diseases. They promise to lower blood pressure and improve cholesterol levels, which means incorporating them into your diet could help safeguard against heart disease (Cassidy et al., 2013).

Now, you might think, *Great. I'll just load up on blueberries then*. But remember, balance is key. While these foods are beneficial, overeating will simply lead to consuming too many calories. Instead of focusing on one superfood, consider creating a colourful plate filled with a variety of fruits and vegetables to confirm you are getting a broad spectrum of nutrients. Sometimes, getting all the required nutrients from food alone may prove unrealistic, given our busy schedules. In such situations, one may rely on high-quality supplements.

Making use of the medicinal properties of food can be really simple. A handful of berries in your morning oatmeal or a side serving of eggplant at dinner can make all the difference. So, how do you incorporate these superfoods into your daily routine? Start by including at least one serving of dark-coloured fruit or vegetable in each meal. Opt for fresh over canned or juiced versions to maximise nutrient content. Consider berries as your snack option instead of processed goods. And remember, consistency is key.

Remember: "Your body hears everything your mind says" (Judd, n.d.). So, nourish it well, not only physically but mentally too. Make informed choices about what you put into your body because, ultimately, these decisions shape how we live our lives—healthy or otherwise.

Key Takeaways

- Processed foods are a major contributor to belly fat. Substituting them with superfoods can result in noticeable fat loss. Some superfoods offer unique compounds that boost metabolism, promote satiety, and limit fat storage.

- Contrary to popular belief, some fats help with fat loss, while certain plant-based foods are protein powerhouses, aiding in satiety and metabolism enhancement.

- Anthocyanins are natural antioxidants found abundantly in red-purple-blue-hued fruits and vegetables with anti-inflammatory properties. It aids in fat loss, healthier body composition, lowers triglyceride levels, improves insulin sensitivity, and promotes overall better health.

- Balance is crucial. Incorporate a variety of nutrient-rich foods into your diet instead of relying solely on one superfood.

- When nutrients are not readily available from the foods you eat, consider high-quality supplements.

Chapter 18:
Meal Planning Strategies for Sustainable Weight Loss

Think of your body as a high-performance vehicle. Just like a car requires the right type of fuel to run efficiently, our bodies need nutritious food to function optimally. Let us start by debunking one common misconception: starving yourself or skipping meals is not the key to fat loss. This approach might show short-term results but can cause long-term damage and lead to an unhealthy relationship with food.

Now, let us delve into how we can plan our meals for sustainable fat loss.

First, whole foods should be prioritised over processed options. Opt for fruits, vegetables, lean proteins, and whole grains. These nutrient-rich choices nourish your body and keep you satisfied for longer. Secondly, mind your portions. Eating the right quantities of food helps nourish your body and also prevents accumulating excess fat. To avoid overeating, consider using smaller plates—research indicates that people consume less when they do so. Thirdly, keep track of what you are eating through a food diary or an app like MyFitnessPal. This practice helps create awareness of what goes into your body and assists in identifying patterns or triggers leading to overeating. Finally, hydration. Drinking plenty of water aids digestion and keeps us feeling full between meals, thus preventing unnecessary snacking.

Remember this quote from Ann Wigmore: "The food you eat can be either the safest and most powerful form of medicine or the slowest form of poison." Let's choose wisely. If belly fat seems stubborn despite regular exercise and balanced dieting, ask healthcare professionals who could provide insights into possible underlying health conditions causing weight retention.

Include fun ways to incorporate healthy eating, such as cooking with family or friends, trying new recipes, or exploring farmers' markets for fresh produce. This makes the journey enjoyable and not just another chore. Meal planning is an effective strategy for sustainable fat loss. It helps us make conscious choices about what we eat and how much we eat. With consistency and patience, this approach can lead us to a healthier future free from the grip of belly fat.

At this stage, I would like to bring to your attention a concerning issue. Over the last 60 years, there has been a decline in the quality and nutrition content of food, especially plant-based food articles. This can be attributed to the adoption of high-yielding varieties of crops, reduced attention to soil management by moving from traditional manures to the chemical enhancement of soils, and atmospheric pollution content. The focus is on quantity rather than quality. The decline has been especially rapid since the green revolution.

Over two billion people suffer from vitamin and mineral deficiencies, especially zinc, vitamin B, vitamin A, and iron. Getting a concentration of nutrients equal to that enjoyed before the pre-green revolution era from food is quite impossible. Profitable crops cultivated on a large scale, like bananas, apples, oranges, mangoes, tomatoes, and potatoes, have lost their nutritional value by up to half over the last five to seven decades. This is caused by a variety of environmental and genetic factors, like deterioration of the soil and genetic modification of the seeds (Bhardwaj et al., 2024).

Global warming also plays a role in the declining nutritional quality of food over time. Food alone may, at times, prove insufficient to meet all the nutritional needs of the body. For example, almost 80% of females do not get the recommended dose of calcium. In such cases, it may be advisable to supplement food with dietary supplements or nutraceuticals, as they are called. These supplements can also specifically target deficiencies without having to unduly pile up calories in the case of elements found only in trace quantities in food.

Some micronutrients are also difficult to absorb or synthesise from food. So, a well-informed choice to depend on supplements from a well-balanced, reputed brand may not be a bad idea. Remember that losing belly fat is not just about looking good; it is about feeling good inside out.

Key Takeaways

- Whole foods over processed foods.
- Portion control matters.
- Keep track of your food intake.
- Stay hydrated.
- Consult healthcare professionals if needed.
- Consider supplements for nutritional deficiencies.

Part V:

Exercise Essentials in Fighting Flab

Chapter 19:
Exercise Basics for Burning Calories Effectively

You don't have to get it perfect; you just have to get it going. Babies do not walk the first time they try, but eventually, they get it right. -Jack Canfield.

A common misconception is that one needs to be a gym rat or run marathons to conquer belly fat. But let us debunk this myth once and for all: moderate exercises with consistency triumph over sporadic bursts of strenuous activities. Think of your body as an engine. We need fuel (food) and maintenance (exercise) to keep the engine running smoothly. Our body keeps burning calories even when it is at rest, referred to as the basal metabolic rate (BMR). This resting metabolic rate is much higher in people with more muscle mass. Hence, every pound of muscle uses about six calories a day just to sustain itself, while each pound of fat burns only two calories daily (Venuto, n.d). The wear and tear of muscles during resistance training also uses up energy for repair. Consistent, moderate exercises can help burn belly fat effectively by increasing our muscle mass and, in turn, our metabolism.

But how does one start building muscles? Let us break this down into simple steps:

- **Step 1: Start small**

Just like trying on a new pair of shoes, your exercise routine should fit you perfectly—not too tight that it hurts, not too loose that it slips off. Start by incorporating small changes, like taking stairs instead of elevators or walking during lunch breaks. Try standing instead of sitting down. Walk while attending calls. Stretching in between bouts of sitting down is a good way to incorporate movement into your daily life.

- **Step 2: Incorporate strength training**

Strength training helps build lean muscle tissues, increasing the resting metabolism rate, leading to calorie burnout even when you are at rest. Now, is that not smart work? Strength training brings to mind big-muscled men lifting heavy weights while grunting and puffing. It does not have to be that strenuous to achieve results. Any movement that contracts muscles against any form of resistance is strength training. This resistance can be from machines at the gym, free weights (like dumbbells, kettlebells, resistance bands, etc.), or even your body weight. Even low-intensity workouts like pilates and yoga can improve strength and muscle mass over time. Ensure that the exercise challenges you. Start with light weights and higher repetitions. This will create the endurance required by the muscles to allow you to exercise for longer without fatigue.

- **Step 3: Cardiovascular Exercises**

This doesn't mean signing up for a marathon immediately. Any activity that gets your heart beating faster counts—dancing, swimming, or even brisk walking. Aim for 30 minutes of moderately intense cardiovascular exercise three times a week. This can be increased as and when you get more comfortable with exercising. Continue for a minimum of three months. The first month can show a dip in weight since you also tend to lose water weight. However, do not expect the weight loss to be as drastic in the following months. The key is to stay committed and consistent with the routine.

What if the problem seems extra bad?

Well, don't lose heart yet. You might want to consider High Intensity Interval Training (HIIT). This involves short bursts of intense workouts followed by short recovery periods. The beauty of HIIT is that it keeps your body burning fat even after you stop exercising. Think of your body working for you while you are binge-watching your favourite Netflix show. HIIT can also be fun and increase functional fitness by allowing you to do normal movements like squatting down, bending, picking up weights, and jumping. The body is designed for movement. Keeping it in motion is a sure way to ensure that it serves you for longer.

However, remember this golden rule: Never let exercise be a punishment for what you ate but a celebration of what your body can do. As we move towards the close of this chapter, let us ponder these words. Exercise because you love yourself and your body and want to take care of it—not because you do not like how it looks.

Remember: consistency over perfection. Let us march forward in our journey towards a healthier self.

Key Takeaways

- Start small and consistent with exercises.
- Incorporate strength training to build lean muscle tissues.
- Cardiovascular activities help burn calories.
- Consider HIIT if the problem seems extra bad.

Chapter 20:
Belly Battles—Specific Exercises for Abdominal Reduction

Going to war with your waistline can feel like a never-ending battle. However, it is not one you are destined to lose. When armed with the right knowledge and strategies, victory is within your reach. Before we delve into the specifics of abdominal exercises, let us step back and look at the battlefield—your belly. Belly fat is more than what meets the eye, as it surrounds vital organs deep inside our body, which makes it particularly dangerous.

Most people think that doing endless crunches will help them get rid of their belly fat, but unfortunately, spot reduction (losing fat from one specific area) is a myth. Exercises that train the muscles in the stomach can definitely strengthen and tone them. However, it does not specifically target the fat within. The body burns fat as a whole rather than from specific areas. So, how do we combat this stubborn belly flab? You need a combination of both cardio (like running or cycling) that burns calories and strength training exercises that build muscle mass since muscles burn more calories even while resting. Studies have shown that high-intensity interval training (HIIT), where you alternate between bursts of intense activity followed by recovery periods, is especially effective in burning abdominal fat (*Belly Fat in Women*, 2023).

Let's look at some practical examples:

1. Planks are great for strengthening your core without adding bulk, making them an excellent part of any belly-fat-busting regimen.

2. Burpees mix strength-building with aerobic conditioning, making them ideal for total-body fitness.

3. Cycling has been proven especially effective at getting rid of visceral (belly) fat because of its cardiovascular nature combined with lower-body resistance training.

4. Swimming works all major muscle groups while providing an aerobic workout, making it an excellent full-body exercise.

Peter Drucker said, "The best way to predict the future is to create it". This quote perfectly encapsulates our approach to belly fat. We are not just passively accepting its presence; we are actively shaping our future by making healthier choices and incorporating effective exercises into our lifestyles.

Let us analyse these exercises more deeply. Planks work by forcing your body—especially your core muscles—to stay in one position for a prolonged period of time. This is referred to as an isometric exercise. Isometric exercises like planks help increase strength, endurance, and stability. Burpees are a dynamic movement that mixes squats, push-ups, and jumps into a potent calorie-burning exercise. Make sure that you work out all major muscle groups of the body. The most important are arms, shoulders, chest, back, and legs. Resistance training has also been found to preserve bone density and reduce age-related muscle wasting. Women especially benefit from resistance training because it protects them against osteoporosis at an advanced age. Cycling and swimming are both low-intensity cardio exercises that help keep those extra pounds away.

The key to losing belly fat and keeping it away is making a lifestyle shift towards staying active. Do not think of exercise as just time spent in your running shoes or on the mat. Incorporate movement into your daily routine. Take breaks and stretch your body in between work at a desk. Try walking while attending calls. Walk to the grocery store instead of taking the car. The human body was built to move. Make small changes to keep the body in motion. Take up exercises you enjoy doing so you can keep up with them. Consistency is key.

Key Takeaways

- Spot reduction is a myth; you need a combination of cardio and strength training exercises for effective belly fat loss.

- Incorporate both resistance training and high-intensity cardio exercises to lose belly fat.

Chapter 21:
How Much Physical Activity Do You Really Need?

There is no one giant step that does it. It's a lot of little steps.

–Peter A. Cohen

When it comes to shedding belly fat, many believe in the misconception that spending countless hours in the gym is the only solution. However, this notion is far from the truth; exercise in moderation, coupled with a suitable diet and lifestyle changes, is key. Think of your body as a car engine that needs regular running for optimal performance. If left idle for long periods, it starts to rust and malfunction. Similarly, our bodies need regular movement to stay healthy and active.

Scientifically speaking, when you engage in physical activity, your body burns calories. The intensity of the exercise determines how many calories you burn. Therefore, if you consume high-calorie food but do not compensate with adequate exercise, these extra calories accumulate as fat deposits around your waistline. As a popular saying goes, "abs are made in the kitchen, not in the gym." Exercising can help tone and strengthen muscles. However, fat can still accumulate in different parts of our body if we continue to eat large amounts of calories that are not commensurate with our physical activity. The amount of energy our bodies expend while resting is called the Basal Metabolic Rate (BMR). Try to keep your calorie intake commensurate with the amount of physical activity you are involved in.

According to the American Heart Association (*American Heart Association*, 2018), adults should aim for at least 30 minutes of moderate-intensity cardiovascular exercise or 15-20 minutes of robust aerobic activity every day. This must be complemented by resistance training for muscle strength and endurance at least twice a week. You could also incorporate low-intensity routines like yoga and pilates to keep the body in motion, get used to movement, and reduce the chance of injury. Understand the limits of your body; pushing it beyond limits can lead to injury, and that would mean periods of inactivity, which would then just be counteractive.

The question then arises: what are moderate-intensity and vigorous-intensity exercises? Think of your workout intensity on a scale from zero to ten, where sitting is zero and working out with the most effort is ten. Moderate-intensity activities would feel like five or six on this scale—activities like brisk walking or light aerobics where you can talk but do not have enough breath to sing. Vigorous workouts clock seven or eight on this scale—these include jogging, running, or swimming laps, where after a few sentences, you would need to catch your breath.

If weight loss appears challenging, consider this: you might be exercising incorrectly. Performing the same workout daily may cause your body to adapt to the routine, reducing its effectiveness over time. Therefore, include a variety of exercises in your fitness regime, like cardio workouts, strength training, and flexibility exercises. For individuals with severe obesity issues or associated health conditions, it is advisable to ask a healthcare professional before starting any exercise plan. They can help devise a suitable exercise regimen based on your physical condition and capabilities.

Remember that Rome was not built in a day. You might not see immediate results, but do not be disheartened; being consistent is the most important component of weight-loss journeys. Take small steps towards adopting healthier habits and gradually progress towards more intense workouts as you build strength and endurance. As Cohen rightly said, "It is all about taking small steps."

Key Takeaways

- Get at least 30 minutes of moderate-intensity cardiovascular exercise or 15-20 minutes of robust aerobic activity every day.
- Incorporate resistance training exercises twice a week.
- Vary your exercises to prevent the body from adapting.
- Consult with healthcare professionals if needed.

Part VI:

Behavioural Changes for Long-Term Success

Chapter 22:
Mindful Eating Techniques to Control Caloric Intake

The secret of change is to focus all your energy on not fighting the old but building new.
-Dan Miller

You probably think you are just eating, and it is a simple, straightforward activity. But have you ever considered the many psychological factors at play while munching on your favourite snack or devouring your dinner? From unconscious snacking in front of the TV to emotional eating, food consumption is a complex process driven by various cognitive and emotional influences. Eating mindfully is an effective strategy for managing your calorie intake, reducing belly fat, and maintaining a healthy weight. Mindful eating entails being completely present during meals, savouring each mouthful, tuning in to hunger cues from your body, and discerning between physical hunger and emotional cravings. It is not about drastic diets or restricting portions; rather, it is about experiencing food more intensely—especially the pleasure of eating itself. You taste every morsel, appreciate its texture, and smell its aroma—all without distractions like television screens or smartphones. This heightened awareness helps you enjoy smaller portions while feeling equally satisfied. Taking time to chew your food properly helps break down the food better and thus aids better digestion.

A study published in Eating Disorders (Kristeller & Wolever, 2010) revealed that people who received mindfulness training experienced significant decreases in stress levels and binge eating episodes compared to those who did not receive such training. This shows evidence of how powerful mindful practices can be when addressing issues related to overeating.

Let us consider Jane as an example. She was always reaching for sugary snacks whenever she felt stressed out at work until she started practising mindful eating techniques. She began acknowledging her feelings instead of resorting to comfort foods and started choosing healthier choices like fruits or nuts when truly hungry.

Analysing these examples provides valuable insights into how changing our habits and practising mindful eating can transform our relationship with food. It is not just about losing belly fat; it is about creating a healthy lifestyle that helps you stay fit in the long run.

In a study published in the Journal of Behavioral Medicine (Godsey, 2017), participants who underwent mindfulness-based interventions showed significant improvements in their eating behaviours, body image perceptions, and emotional well-being compared to those who did not participate in such programmes.

Mindfulness-based interventions most commonly centre on yoga, meditation, cognitive therapy, and eating awareness training. Mindfulness encourages individuals to understand the experience and expression of emotions so they can identify and challenge their beliefs and attend and respond to their feelings adaptively instead of turning to maladaptive practices like overeating. Mindful eating also helps to remove judgement and guilt associated with eating and experience it as an enjoyable emotion. Remember, mindful eating is not a replacement for other measures to cut down abdominal obesity. It needs to be used in conjunction with a balanced diet and continuous physical activity to reap maximum benefit.

Here are some interesting points about mindful eating:

- It promotes self-awareness about physical hunger and satiety cues.

- It slows down the pace of your meals, which can lead to a lower calorie intake.

- This technique encourages appreciation for quality over quantity of food.

According to a report by Harvard Health Publishing (*Mindful Eating*, 2011), mindful eating has been associated with fat loss, improved psychological health, reduced binge-eating episodes, decreased depressive symptoms, and increased self-confidence.

Now let's get into specific steps you need to take for successful implementation of this practice:

1. Sit down and eliminate distractions: Make every meal an event. Sit at a table without distractions like TV or smartphones so that you can focus solely on your meal.

2. Eat slowly: Take smaller portions of food per bite and chew deliberately. Savour each mouthful before swallowing it; this will also help the digestion process by better breaking down the food before reaching your stomach.

3. Listen to your body signals: Recognise when you're hungry and when you are full; stop eating once you feel satisfied, even if there is still food left on your plate.

4. Appreciate your food: Think about where the food came from, how it was grown, and who prepared it. This will help you feel more connected to your meal.

5. Practice gratitude: Start each meal with a moment of appreciation. Appreciate the nourishment your food provides.

Begin implementing these steps in your daily routine and experience noticeable changes in your eating habits; reducing belly fat will just be an added bonus.

Key Takeaways

- Mindful eating encourages conscious awareness during mealtimes, leading to healthier food choices and controlled caloric intake.

- Mindfulness techniques can noticeably improve your attitude towards food, leading to healthier habits.

- Slowing down and savouring each bite makes meals more satisfying and helps control portion sizes.

- Practising mindful eating can offer numerous health benefits beyond weight reduction alone.

Chapter 23:
Building Resilience Towards Food Cravings

As we embark on this journey, let me assure you that the fight against belly fat is not just about physical exercises and dieting; it is equally about behaviour change. In my many years of studying and researching this subject, I have come across fascinating insights into our relationship with food. Did you know that our brain is wired to crave high-calorie foods? It harks back to our ancestors, who needed calorie-dense foods for survival. Today, however, these cravings can lead to unhealthy eating habits and consequent belly fat accumulation.

Now onto the meatier part of the discussion. To successfully maintain a healthy waistline in the long run, we need a strategic approach that involves understanding food cravings, identifying triggers, and building resilience towards them. Scientific evidence backs this up. A study published in Frontiers in Psychology (RodrÃguez-MartÃn & Meule, 2015) found that people who understand their cravings are more successful at managing them compared to those who simply try to suppress or ignore them.

Let us consider Jane's story as an example here. Jane was a habitual snack eater who could not resist her evening cookie-jar visits. However, when she began noting down what she was doing each time these cravings hit her, she realised most of her snacking happened while watching TV after dinner. Identifying such triggers helped Jane replace her snacking habit with walking during commercial breaks instead.

As motivational speaker Brian Tracy once said, "The ability to discipline yourself to delay gratification in the short term to enjoy greater rewards in the long term is the indispensable prerequisite for success." There is no magic pill that will help you reduce that stubborn fat accumulating around your waist. It is all about small and consistent steps towards the goal of a healthier lifestyle. Drastic diets and completely eliminating certain food groups or macronutrients do little to set you on the path to long-term health. It boils down to moderation and sustained effort. Choose small healthy habits like sleeping on time, eating small and less processed meals at fixed times during the day, moving your body every day, and meditating for a couple of minutes. These basic changes go a long way towards bringing about huge changes in the long run.

Analysing your triggers helps create effective strategies against unhealthy eating patterns that lead directly to belly fat accumulation. One compelling case study comes from a research paper published by Integrative Medicine (Cherpak, 2019). The researchers observed participants over six months as they implemented mindfulness techniques to understand their eating triggers. The results showed an impressive reduction in binge-eating instances and overall fat loss. Train your body to stop eating when your stomach feels three-fourths full. This can aid digestion and can also keep you feeling light and energetic. This is an effective way to restrict those calories that we unnecessarily put into our bodies while trying to polish off our plates.

Some interesting points to note:

- Cravings are not just influenced by physical hunger but by emotional states as well.

- Distractions like TV or work can lead to mindless eating.

- Sugary and fatty foods tend to be the most craved items.

Statistics from the CDC show that over 42% of American adults are obese, a crisis largely attributed to unhealthy eating patterns (*Prevalence of Overweight*, 2019). Furthermore, research shows that a persistent pattern of overeating increases belly fat accumulation significantly.

Now, let us get down to some actionable steps you can take today:

1. Understand Your Cravings: Start noting when your cravings hit. What were you doing? How were you feeling?

2. Identify triggers: Are there specific activities or emotions associated with your cravings? Minimise these triggers where possible.

3. Practise mindful eating: Pay attention while you eat, savour each bite, and avoid distractions during mealtimes.

4. Replace Bad Habits with Good Ones: If TV time equals snack time for you, try replacing it with something healthier like a walk or reading a book instead.

5. Practice meditation to eliminate stress and to be able to cope with difficult emotions constructively rather than turn to maladaptive coping mechanisms.

6. Get a medical check-up to rule out any deficiencies that could be causing the cravings.

With this knowledge at your disposal and the right mindset, I believe anyone can build resilience against food cravings and pave their way towards long-term success against belly fat.

Key Takeaways

- Understanding your food cravings is key to managing them effectively.

- Mindfulness techniques can help manage food cravings effectively.

- Identifying your personal triggers is fundamental to managing food cravings.

- Unhealthy eating patterns directly contribute to obesity and belly fat accumulation.

Chapter 24:
Motivation Maintenance Strategies for Consistent Efforts

A pathway of a thousand miles begins with a single step, and the same applies to your belly fat loss. It is like climbing a mountain; it seems intimidating at first, but once you start moving upwards, there is no turning back. The real challenge, however, is not taking the first step or reaching the top but maintaining consistent efforts throughout.

One fine day, you decide to lose that stubborn belly fat and make lifestyle changes like eating healthy and exercising regularly. But your motivation dwindles as days turn into weeks and weeks into months. You start craving those sugary treats again or skipping workouts because of exhaustion from work. Losing belly fat becomes an uphill battle against two formidable enemies: laziness and a lack of discipline. But do not worry. This chapter will equip you with effective motivational strategies so your path towards a flat belly and a healthier life stays steady.

- Understanding why you started: Remembering why you initially decided to shed that extra weight can serve as a powerful motivator. Write down your reasons—be it health concerns or aesthetic desires—on sticky notes around your house or set reminders on your phone.

- Setting realistic goals: Set achievable goals rather than aspiring for drastic changes overnight. Celebrate small victories, like choosing salad over pizza or walking instead of driving to nearby places.

- Making healthy habits fun: Find ways to incorporate fun into achieving your targets. For example, dance while cooking healthy meals or listen to an audiobook while jogging.

Failure is part of any journey, including losing weight. If one day you end up eating more than the required calories or missing workouts because of unavoidable circumstances, do not beat yourself up. Instead, rise again and continue your journey. Do not think of it as a means to an end. Learn to enjoy the process of eating healthy and staying active. Keep track of your progress to stay motivated and make more gains. Partner up with a friend or family member so they keep you accountable for the progress. Having a mentor, coach, or friend makes it easier to keep you focused on the shift you are trying to make.

For those struggling with extreme weight issues, it is advisable to seek professional help from dietitians or fitness trainers who can provide customised plans based on personal needs. Consulting a professional is similar to having a GPS while trekking; it guides you in the right direction when you feel lost. It also helps to draw on the experiences of multiple other people who have gone through similar problems and have emerged successful in overcoming them.

Remember, motivation is not constant but fluctuating. Staying motivated throughout is challenging but crucial for long-term success in losing belly fat. With these strategies at hand, keep going strong towards your goal.

Key Takeaways

- Identify why you want to lose belly fat.
- Break your long-term goals into small achievable tasks and celebrate small victories.
- Make your healthy habits fun and enjoyable.
- Seek professional help if required.

Part VII:

Living Young & Aging Healthy

Chapter 25:
Anti-Ageing Secrets and Belly Fat—The Undeniable Connection

You might not see it yet, but there is a startling connection between belly fat and ageing. It goes beyond the surface-level changes we often associate with growing older; those extra pounds around your midsection can have profound implications for your overall health and longevity. Belly fat is a harbinger of potential health issues. Adipose tissue will often attach to vital organs, leading to the risk of chronic metabolic diseases like coronary disease, kidney problems, and diabetes. (*Abdominal Fat*, 2019). Worse still, it has been linked to premature ageing. For years, scientists have been researching the link between excess body weight and accelerated ageing processes. They have uncovered that belly fat contributes to inflammation in the body, which can damage cells' functionality over time—akin to rusting from within.

Now let us unravel this complex issue together.

In my experience working with clients struggling with weight issues, I've found that understanding is half the battle. When you understand how belly fat accelerates ageing and jeopardises your health, you are more likely to take meaningful action towards fighting it off. The evidence supporting these claims is robust. In one study by the Mayo Clinic (Cerhan et al., 2014), researchers showed that participants with larger waistlines had shorter life expectancies regardless of their overall body mass index (BMI). Another study published in The Lancet found that abdominal obesity was strongly linked with higher mortality rates (Tobias & Hu, 2018).

Let us consider some real-life examples too. Think about people around you who lead sedentary lifestyles or have unhealthy eating habits; they tend to age faster compared to those who exercise regularly and eat nutritious food.

Bethenny Frankel, founder and CEO of Skinnygirl, once said, "Your diet is a bank account. Good food choices are good investments." This quote is a simple yet profound reminder that our food choices directly impact our health and longevity. Analysing the belly fat problem provides us with an actionable solution: adopting a healthier lifestyle. This includes staying physically active, eating a balanced diet, getting sufficient sleep, and managing stress effectively. Case studies have repeatedly shown the effectiveness of these changes. A study published in Obesity Reviews found that combining dietary modifications with regular physical activity resulted in significant reductions in belly fat among participants (Brown et al., 2009).

Here are some interesting bullet points to consider regarding abdominal fat and ageing:

- Belly fat produces inflammatory substances that can damage cells.

- Regular exercise helps reduce inflammation and improve cell function.

- A balanced diet rich in fibre, protein, fruits, and vegetables reduces the risk of excess belly fat accumulation.

- Minimise use of alcohol, cigarettes, and other intoxicants.

Advancing age increases the probability of chronic diseases such as stroke, heart disease, and diabetes. Accompanying ageing is also the increase in white adipose tissues (the energy-storing fat found in our tummies.), which further increases the risk for such diseases (Brown et al., 2009).

Diet and behaviour therapy have been found to reduce the risk of breast cancer recurrence at 5 years and ovarian cancer in the final 4 years of an 8-year trial. Low-fat diets can reduce type 2 diabetes, improve blood pressure, and reduce antihypertensive medication for up to 3 years. Diet and exercise reduce the risk of type 2 diabetes for up to 6 years and metabolic syndrome at 4 years, compared with control groups. However, a non-reducing diet and behaviour therapy did not reduce diabetes risk in nearly 49,000 women after 8.1 years. The model predicted that the intervention estimated a survival of 0.18 years (Brown et al., 2009).

As for specific action steps you can take:

Start by incorporating more physical activity into your day—even brisk walking for half an hour daily can make a difference. Gradually introduce strength training exercises into your routine to build muscle mass, which burns calories more effectively than body fat does.

Rethink your eating habits, too. Prioritise whole foods over processed ones, and increase your intake of lean proteins while reducing excessive sugars and unhealthy fats. Lastly, confirm you are getting enough rest each night, as inadequate sleep has been linked to weight gain. Remember, these changes do not need to be drastic or immediate; small, consistent steps can lead to big changes over time.

To wrap up this chapter, let us remember that our health is an investment—one that requires not only financial resources but also time, effort, and dedication. And it is absolutely worth it because, at the end of the day, what matters more than living young and dying healthy?

Key Takeaways

- Belly fat is more than just an aesthetic problem; it poses significant risks for chronic diseases and accelerates ageing.

- Adopting a healthier lifestyle is one of the most effective ways to fight off belly fat and slow down ageing.

- Inflammation caused by belly fat can be mitigated through regular exercise and a balanced diet.

- The global obesity epidemic emphasises the importance of addressing belly fat accumulation at personal and societal levels.

Chapter 26:

How to Achieve a Healthy Lifestyle for Longevity

Take care of your body—it's the only place you have to live.

–Jim Rohn

It is a beautiful day, is it not? Let us start our conversation with that fresh energy. You have learned about belly fat, why we get it, the dangers it poses, and how to lose it sustainably. Today, we'll talk about achieving a healthy lifestyle for longevity. Have you ever wondered why some people seem ageless? They are vibrant, full of life, and brimming with health well into their later years. It is not just genetics; lifestyle plays a pivotal role too.

When we speak of living young and dying healthy, we are talking about more than just maintaining an ideal body weight or staying free from disease. We are talking about holistic health—physical activity, balanced nutrition, quality sleep—and psychological wellness—stress management and positive social relationships.

Over the years, I have discovered something interesting: The key to ageing gracefully is adopting healthy habits early on that can last a lifetime—an active lifestyle combined with good nutrition.

Research shows that exercise has profound effects on our mental health by reducing symptoms of depression and anxiety while improving cognitive function. Regular physical activity keeps your heart strong—a kind of "fountain of youth" for your heart—and helps control blood pressure levels. Nutritionally speaking, aim to consume whole foods rich in antioxidants like fruits and vegetables—they help combat free radicals, which are responsible for ageing. Also, include lean proteins for muscle repair or growth as you age; omega-3 fatty acids found in fish oils boost brain health; fibre keeps your digestive system running smoothly; calcium and vitamin D ensure bone strength; probiotics enhance gut health—the list goes on.

This quote sums up our discussion quite well. Your body is your home, and taking care of it now ensures you reap the benefits in later years.

Looking at belly fat from a new angle, we see that it's not just about appearance or self-esteem; it is a serious health concern. It can lead to conditions like heart disease, diabetes, and even certain cancers. By sustaining healthy habits over time—like regular exercise and balanced nutrition—you'll be reducing these risks substantially.

One study showed that people who maintained five healthy lifestyle factors—never smoking, maintaining a healthy weight, regular physical activity, moderate alcohol consumption, and consuming a nutritious diet—lived more than 14 years longer on average than those who did not maintain any of these behaviours (Li et al., 2018). Having a daily routine can help build a healthy lifestyle. Have fixed sleep schedules and incorporate exercise into your daily routine.

In cases of specific deficiencies, supplements are considered for management. Opt for high-quality supplements backed by scientific, evidence-based research. The nutrition profile of food has deteriorated in the last couple of decades. The nutrition you got from one head of broccoli can now be obtained by consuming almost three heads of broccoli. Supplements can fill these gaps and provide the body with exactly the doses of nutrients needed to keep it young. It can also help in tackling the free radical exposure that the body is exposed to in so many different forms in today's world.

Here are some actionable steps for you:

1. Regular exercise: Start with simple workouts like walking or yoga, then gradually increase intensity as your fitness improves.

2. Balanced nutrition: Incorporate whole foods into your meals while minimising processed food intake.

3. Adequate sleep: Aim for 7-9 hours per night to allow your body to recover.

4. Stress management: Practice mindfulness techniques like meditation or deep breathing exercises.

5. Positive social relationships: Maintain good relationships with family and friends—it contributes significantly to mental health.

6. Consider supplements: If food alone is unable to eliminate all deficiencies, supplements can be a good choice.

Summarising the findings of the 2018 study by Li et al.:

- Physical Activity + Balanced Nutrition = Reduced Belly Fat

- Reduced Belly Fat + Healthy Lifestyle = Increased Longevity

The World Health Organization found that physical inactivity is the fourth major risk factor for mortality across the globe, responsible for an estimated 3 million deaths (World Obesity Day, 2022). Longevity does not happen overnight; start small and be consistent. You have taken the first step by educating yourself about belly fat; now it is time to put that knowledge into action. Remember, it is never too late to start living young and dying healthy.

Key Takeaways

- Longevity is not merely about living longer but also about living healthier.

- Adopting healthier lifestyle choices promotes longevity.

- The formula for living young and dying healthy involves adopting an active lifestyle combined with good nutrition and other wellness practices.

- Regular physical activity reduces the risk of many adverse health outcomes.

Chapter 27:
Importance of Regular Health Check-Ups

Ageing is an inevitable part of life, but that does not mean we have to resign ourselves to a future filled with ailments and declining health. You have heard the saying, "Prevention is better than cure." Well, it is not just a cliché; it is scientific truth.

Imagine you are driving a car. You take it for regular servicing to confirm its smooth operation, right? Our bodies are no different. They need regular 'servicing' in the form of health check-ups.

A study published by Li et al. (2018) affirms this analogy by stating that people who go for routine medical screening have a 24% lower risk of premature death compared to those who do not. Regular check-ups can nip potential health issues in the bud before they grow into full-blown problems. It is like having your personal team of detectives on hand, ready to catch any villains trying to sabotage your health. There are micronutrients that your body needs to keep functioning optimally. Inadequacies, if any, in the micronutrient profile can be detected by timely health check-ups.

Here is something interesting from Dr. Robert Butler, Pulitzer Prize-winning author and former director of the National Institute on Ageing: "I decided that doctors do all they can to keep people alive and give them the best possible life, so I made up my mind I was going to be a doctor" (*Robert N. Butler, 2020*).

These words resonate because they emphasise how important regular interactions with healthcare professionals are when aiming for longevity and good health.

Step-by-step guide on how you can make these health check-ups a part of your life:

1. Start with an annual physical examination. This includes basic measurements (height, weight), checking vital signs (blood pressure, heart rate), blood tests, etc., essentially giving an overall view of your physical status.

2. Go for Routine Blood Tests: These tests provide insights about cholesterol levels (linked directly with belly fat), sugar levels, etc., helping watch conditions like diabetes or cardiovascular diseases closely.

3. Never skip your dental check-ups: Oral health is often an overlooked aspect of overall well-being. Regular dental check-ups can prevent gum disease and tooth decay.

4. Get regular eye examinations. They not only confirm good vision but also help identify early signs of conditions like glaucoma or macular degeneration.

5. Prioritise Mental Health Check-ups: Mental health is as important as physical health, and regular counselling sessions or mental health screenings can do wonders for your overall well-being.

If you are worried about the time commitment, think about this: What is a few hours every year compared to adding years to your life?

Remember, it is not just about extending our lives but also enhancing their quality. So, embrace these regular 'servicing' appointments with a smile, and let us live young and die healthy.

Key Takeaways

- Regular health check-ups are crucial for the early detection and prevention of diseases.

- Making healthcare professionals your allies in the journey towards healthy living is essential.

- Your annual schedule should include routine blood tests, eye exams, dental check-ups, and mental health screenings.

Part VIII:

Managing Weight in Different Life Stages

Chapter 28:
Losing Baby Weight—Post-Pregnancy Waistline Woes

As a new mom, you may find yourself grappling with a list of novel challenges and changes that your body has undergone. One such change that often causes distress is the stubborn belly fat that seems to have made itself quite at home during pregnancy. Do not worry. You are not alone in this battle.

Belly fat post-pregnancy is undeniably common, and it is not just about aesthetics. The reason why it is so hard to lose is because the body stores excess energy as visceral fat around the abdomen area. This accumulation happens because of hormonal changes during pregnancy, which make your body store more fat as a buffer for breastfeeding. It is nature's way of ensuring there are enough energy reserves for both mom and baby.

But why does it seem easier for some women to lose baby weight than others? It all comes down to genetics, lifestyle factors, diet habits, and exercise regimens. Scientific evidence supports these claims too. One study conducted by researchers from University College London found that pregnant women who ate a high-sugar and high-fibre diet were less likely to retain postnatal weight than those who consumed diets low in fibre or high in glycaemic load (foods that quickly raise blood sugar) (Drehmer et al., 2012).

So, now we know what triggers belly fat retention after pregnancy. But how do we combat it?

Firstly, let's debunk one myth: crash diets don't work. They may show results initially, but they are not sustainable, long-term solutions. It could also leave you feeling drained and not up for the new challenges of motherhood. It is very important to stay positive and energetic even as you try to shed those excess pounds. Instead, focus on nourishing your body with balanced meals packed full of vegetables, lean proteins, healthy fats, and complex carbohydrates.

Secondly, introduce regular physical activity into your routine. This doesn't mean you should jump straight into high-intensity workouts. Start with moderate exercises such as brisk walking or light aerobics, and gradually increase intensity over time. If possible, try to involve your child or partner while working out to make it more enjoyable and sustainable. Remember, the goal is not just to lose weight but to improve overall health and fitness levels.

Analysing these steps, it is clear that losing baby weight is more about making lifestyle adjustments than turning to drastic measures. It is about creating a sustainable routine that you can keep up with even in changing circumstances. Remember that the few extra pounds will eventually come off as you nurse your newborn and get back to a stress-free routine. Keep in mind that your body has been through a stressful period and that it needs time to get back to feeling like before pregnancy. Be patient and gradual with your physical activity.

Several case studies highlight the effectiveness of this approach. For instance, a study published in the Journal of Women's Health found that women who followed diet and exercise interventions after pregnancy were more successful at losing weight than those who didn't (O'Toole et al., 2003).

Interesting points:

- Hormonal changes during pregnancy contribute to belly fat.

- Genes, diet habits, and physical activity also play a role.

- Crash diets aren't effective, long-term solutions.

- Gradually increasing physical activity aids in weight loss.

- Aim for overall health improvement rather than just shedding pounds.

Another important aspect is stress management. High levels of stress can trigger cortisol production, which may lead to increased appetite and, therefore, weight gain. Therefore, incorporating stress-relieving activities like yoga or meditation into your routine can be useful. According to the Centers for Disease Control and Prevention (Cramer, 2016), most women retain an average of one to six pounds one year after giving birth, while around half of all pregnant women gain more weight than the recommended guidelines suggest during their pregnancies.

So, how do you get started? Here are some specific steps:

1. Start with balanced meals: Include a variety of fruits, vegetables, whole grains, lean proteins, and healthy fats in your diet.

2. Gradually increase physical activity: Begin with light exercises like walking or yoga and slowly raise intensity over time.

3. Manage stress: Incorporate relaxation techniques into your routine to keep cortisol levels under control.

Remember, everyone's journey is unique, and what works for you may not work for another. Listen to your body and consult health professionals if needed.

Key Takeaways

- Belly fat post-pregnancy is common, but losing it can be challenging because of hormonal changes and lifestyle factors.

- Sustainable lifestyle changes are key to losing post-pregnancy belly fat.

- Stress management plays an essential role in managing post-pregnancy belly fat.

- Weight retention after pregnancy is common but can be managed through sustainable lifestyle modifications.

Chapter 29:
Dealing With Midlife Metabolism Slowdown

As we age, it is as if our bodies start to play a cruel joke on us. We continue to eat the same amount of food and engage in the same activities, but suddenly, that dreaded belly fat begins to appear. It is like an unwanted guest who overstays their welcome at a party. You might be wondering, *Why am I gaining weight when I am not eating any differently?* The answer comes from your metabolism.

Think of your metabolism as a fiery furnace. In our youth, this furnace is blazing hot; it burns everything we throw into it quickly and efficiently. But come midlife, the fire starts flickering; it no longer burns as fiercely. This slowdown is often referred to as a 'midlife metabolic slowdown'.

But fear not. There are ways to rekindle this metabolic fire and keep that unwelcome belly fat at bay.

Age-related weight gain is not inevitable. Understanding your changing metabolism can help you adjust your lifestyle habits and keep weight gain under control.

One might ask, Why does our metabolism slow down with age? As we get older, we tend to lose muscle mass because of decreased activity levels or hormonal changes. Muscle cells need more energy than fat cells do, even when they're not being used. So, having fewer muscle cells means you'll burn fewer calories and store more fat. To combat this problem, consider taking up strength training exercises that help build muscle mass while also boosting your metabolic rate, even when you are resting.

In addition to exercise adjustments, diet plays a crucial role too. Refined carbs and sugary foods may have been easier for young metabolisms to handle but will likely linger longer in older bodies, leading to weight gain. Instead, focus on consuming lean proteins such as chicken or tofu, which take longer for the body to digest, thereby keeping you satiated for longer periods while also requiring more energy to process.

And then there is the importance of sleep. Lack of sleep can disrupt your metabolism and lead to weight gain. So, make sure you are getting plenty of rest each night. It is important to remember that midlife is not a death sentence for your waistline. As George Eliot once said, "It is never too late to be what you might have been."

If Things Are Extra Bad?

For those who may be facing severe weight issues related to midlife metabolic slowdown, consider seeking professional help from a dietician or a health coach. Invasive medical interventions such as bariatric surgery should be considered only in extreme cases, as there can be downstream complications if not managed properly. Remember, the body is a wonder machine capable of self-healing much more than we give it credit for. The better you take care of it, the better it will serve you.

Key Takeaways

- Midlife metabolic slowdown: Your metabolism slows down as you age, leading to potential weight gain.

- Exercise: Strength training exercises can boost your metabolism by building muscle mass.

- Diet: Opt for lean proteins and cut down on refined carbs and sugary foods.

- Sleep: A good night's rest is essential for maintaining healthy metabolic functions.

- It's never too late: Age-related weight gain isn't inevitable. Changes in diet, activity levels, and lifestyle habits can help manage your body's changing needs.

Remember, this journey is not about achieving an 'ideal' body but ensuring that we provide our bodies with the best possible care at every stage of life.

Chapter 30:
Elderly and Obesity—Special Considerations

Age is no barrier. It's a limitation you put on your mind. -Jackie Joyner-Kersee

The autumn season of life, often known as old age, is a time when the body starts showing signs of wear and tear. One such manifestation is weight gain, specifically around the midsection. Belly fat in the elderly poses a unique set of health risks that are not only different but also more severe than those faced by younger people.

Belly fat is not just an aesthetic issue; it is a ticking time bomb for numerous health problems like heart disease, diabetes, and even certain types of cancer. As you age, your metabolism naturally slows down, making losing weight harder. Plus, with retirement often comes decreased physical activity, which can further contribute to weight gain. Interestingly enough, elderly adults have an entirely different type of belly fat than their younger counterparts. It is called visceral fat, and it wraps itself around your internal organs like a snug blanket on a cold winter's night. This makes it even more dangerous because it can interfere with how your organs function.

Now, let's explore this problem more deeply and talk about some solutions.

Regular exercise is essential to controlling belly fat at any age but particularly critical for seniors because of its myriad benefits: improved heart health, increased flexibility and balance (thus reducing the risk of falls), better sleep quality, and mood regulation.

But here's the catch: given their physical limitations or pre-existing medical conditions, elderly individuals may find traditional workouts challenging or even impossible. So, what should they do? Here is where low-impact exercises come in handy—think yoga or tai chi. These forms of exercise are gentle on joints yet effective in burning calories.

A study in The American Journal of Clinical Nutrition found that yoga helped reduce waist circumference among elderly women (Cramer, 2016). Take the case of 75-year-old Martha Stewart. The lifestyle guru swears by yoga and a healthy diet to maintain her age-defying physique and vibrant energy. Her example illustrates how taking control of belly fat is possible and rewarding at an older age (Dyett, 2022).

Analysing this issue further, we find that it's not just physical activity that matters but also what you eat. As metabolism slows with age, so does the calorie requirement, which means seniors need fewer calories than before.

A study published in The Journal of Nutrition Health & Aging confirmed that a Mediterranean-style diet rich in fruits, vegetables, lean proteins, whole grains, and healthy fats can help manage weight and improve overall health among elderly adults (Zbeida et al., 2014).

Here are some facts for thought:

- According to the Centers for Disease Control (CDC), nearly 40% of Americans aged 60 or older were obese as of 2016 (*Prevalence of Overweight*, 2019).

- Research shows people aged 60 or older need about 200 fewer calories per day compared to their younger selves because of their slower metabolism (Callahan, 2020).

To combat belly fat effectively:

1. Follow a regular exercise routine comprising gentle yet effective workouts like tai chi or yoga.

2. Adopt a healthier eating pattern, favouring whole foods over processed ones.

3. Regularly watch your weight and make necessary modifications along the way.

4. Consult your healthcare provider before starting any new fitness regimen or making drastic dietary changes, especially if you have pre-existing medical conditions.

These steps might seem daunting at first, but remember, it is never too late to make positive changes. Your golden years are meant to be enjoyed in good health and in high spirits. So, take that first step today towards a healthier you.

Key Takeaways

- Regular, low-impact exercise helps burn calories and manage belly fat without straining the joints.

- A balanced diet low in processed foods and high in nutrient-dense ones aids weight management and boosts overall health.

- Ageing naturally lowers the metabolic rate, leading to lower calorie requirements, thus making dietary adjustments necessary for weight management.

Part IX:

Overcoming Obstacles in Your Fitness Journey

Chapter 31:
Plateauing—When the Scale Doesn't Budge Anymore

The fitness journey is filled with ups and downs. You might be cruising along, watching the numbers on the scale decline week after week until suddenly they stop. Despite doing everything right in your nutrition and exercise plan, you have hit a plateau. This chapter will help you understand why plateaus happen and how to overcome them.

Plateaus are not unusual in any fitness journey; they are just your body's way of saying it is become too comfortable with its current routine. Your body is an incredible machine designed for survival, constantly adapting to make things easier for itself. So, when you continually do the same exercises or eat the same amount of calories, your body gets used to it and responds by burning fewer calories. Understanding this can be both fascinating and frustrating. On one hand, it shows our bodies' amazing ability to adapt, but on the other hand, it also means progress is not always linear. But do not despair. Hitting a plateau does not mean that you have failed or that losing more weight is impossible. It just means that something has to change.

One study published in the Journal of Clinical Endocrinology & Metabolism found that dieters who had hit a plateau were able to start losing weight again after changing their calorie intake or exercise routine. The researchers concluded that changes in either energy input (calories consumed) or output (calories burned) could disrupt the plateau effect (Sumithran et al., 2011). For example, if you have been running three miles every day at the same pace since starting your fitness journey, try adding some variety to your workout regime, like incorporating sprints or hill runs instead of only doing steady-state cardio all the time.

Overcoming plateaus involves persisting through those frustrating moments and making the necessary changes to keep moving forward. Solving your plateau problem might include changing your diet, tweaking your exercise routine, or even adjusting your sleep and stress levels. It is all about finding a new balance that will force your body to adapt once again. Fall in love with your exercise routine. Do not see exercise as a punishment for all the calories consumed.

Consider the story of Sarah, who was featured in "The New York Times" for her fat-loss journey. After losing 50 pounds, she hit a plateau that lasted several months. She could not understand why until her nutritionist pointed out that she was consuming too many hidden calories in her supposedly healthy smoothies. By replacing them with protein-rich snacks instead, Sarah overcame her plateau and continued losing weight (Miller, 2020).

The most important aspect to keep in mind is not to stress out or despair. Take it in stride and try to seek logical solutions rationally. Make sure your food portions are in place, that you are getting physical activity, that you are sleeping well, and that you are in a positive frame of mind. All these contribute to having a wholesome weight management journey. Stress and cortisol have been found to have an impact on the fat that accumulates in the abdominal cavity. Make sure you are consistent in your approach and that you are not resorting to extreme or fad measures. The easier it is to follow, the more consistent your results will be. Try to remember that we want to enjoy the process because fitness is never an end goal. If we view it as one end goal, it is easy to fall back into old routines and thus lose all the gains.

Some interesting points:

- You don't necessarily have to work harder or eat less when you hit a plateau; sometimes you just need to work differently.

- Changing up both diet and exercise routines is often more effective than focusing on one aspect alone.

- Even small changes can make a big difference in disrupting the plateau effect.

According to data from the National Weight Control Registry (NWCR), individuals who successfully maintain long-term fat loss often use strategies such as varying their diet and exercise routines, consistently tracking their progress, and seeking support from others when they hit a plateau (Klem et al., 1997).

Here are some specific steps you can take:

1. Evaluate your diet: Are there any hidden sources of calories or sugar? Could you be eating larger portions than necessary?

2. Change your exercise routine: Try a new type of workout, increase the intensity or frequency, or add resistance training if you have not already.

3. Monitor your progress: Regularly track your weight, body measurements, and other indicators of health to see if changes are happening, even if they are not reflected on the scale.

4. Seek support: Don't hesitate to ask for help from a fitness professional or join a support group. Sometimes an outside perspective can identify what you might be missing.

Remember that overcoming plateaus is part of the process. It is not always straightforward, but with perseverance and adaptability, you'll keep moving towards your fitness goals.

Key Takeaways

- Plateauing happens when your body adapts to its current routine; change is necessary for further progress.

- Hidden factors can cause plateaus; it's essential to examine all aspects of your lifestyle.

- Small changes can lead to significant results in overcoming plateaus.

- Regular monitoring of progress and variety in routines are common strategies among successful long-term weight-lossers.

Chapter 32:

Bouncing Back From Failures and Setbacks

Every journey has its ups and downs, including your fitness journey. The road to a healthier you is filled with many obstacles, some of which may seem insurmountable. You might fall off the wagon or hit a plateau that feels like an impenetrable wall. But remember, as famous scientist Albert Einstein once said, "You never fail until you stop trying." Let us begin this chapter by visualising our fitness journey as climbing up a mountain. The higher we climb, the more challenging it gets because of thinning oxygen levels (more challenges), slippery slopes (unexpected setbacks), and harsh weather conditions (external factors). Just like on a real mountain expedition, preparation, persistence, and resilience are key.

But what happens when we lose our footing?

1. Acknowledge your feelings

Firstly, when you experience failure or setbacks in your fat loss goal—perhaps you have gained back some pounds after indulging during the holidays—do not ignore your feelings. Feeling disappointed or frustrated is okay; it means you care about your progress.

2. Reflect on what went wrong

Next comes reflection: understanding why the slip-up happened in the first place—were there triggers? Did stress push you towards comfort eating? Understanding these patterns can help prevent future derailments.

3. Reset Your perspective

Remember that setbacks are not permanent unless we allow them to be; they are merely detours in your path, not the end of it. Forgive yourself for any mistakes made and reset your perspective by focusing on how far you've come rather than dwelling on temporary failures.

4. Have a Plan B

125

Always have strategies ready for unexpected hurdles, whether it's having healthy snacks available when cravings hit or finding indoor workout options for rainy days.

5. Get back on track

The key to bouncing back is not giving up. Get back on track with your healthy eating and exercise routine as soon as you can.

If the problem seems extra bad, for instance, if you are unable to stop binge eating or if working out consistently seems impossible because of a busy schedule, consider seeking professional help. A registered dietitian can provide personalised guidance, while a fitness trainer can create an exercise plan that fits into your hectic life.

Remember, every failure carries with it the seed of equal or greater success. Your ability to bounce back from setbacks determines the extent of your achievement in this journey towards losing belly fat and gaining a healthier lifestyle. Overcoming obstacles in your fitness journey is more about mental strength than physical capability. With persistence and resilience, you'll find that every setback brings you one step closer to reaching the peak of your personal 'fitness mountain'.

Key Takeaways

- Acknowledge your feelings when experiencing setbacks.
- Reflect on what went wrong and learn from it.
- Reset your perspective; focus on progress over perfection.
- Have backup strategies ready for unexpected hurdles.
- Get back on track as soon as possible.

Chapter 33:
Preparing for Unexpected Changes and Challenges

Obstacles don't have to stop you. If you run into a wall, don't turn around and give up. Figure out how to climb it. -Michael Jordan

In the journey towards maintaining a healthy body and losing belly fat, it is crucial to anticipate that there will be obstacles along the way. You have probably heard of Murphy's Law: if anything can go wrong, it will. Well, in fitness, too, life may throw curveballs at you. It might be an injury or an unexpected event disrupting your routine. But do not worry. With some knowledge and planning, you can navigate these hurdles gracefully.

Many years ago, when I started my fitness journey, no one told me that there would be various hitches down the road. The truth is that change is inevitable in life; hence, your fitness journey won't always be smooth sailing either. The first step to overcoming obstacles on this path is acknowledging their existence. Once you are aware of potential pitfalls, you can prepare accordingly and minimise their impact on your progress. In all my years as a health coach, I have seen countless instances where unforeseen circumstances disrupted people's routines, leading to frustration and demotivation. That is why we are going to delve into strategies for dealing with such situations effectively.

Evidence shows that those who maintain long-term fat loss adapt well to changes (Wing & Phelan, 2005). These individuals do not let disruptions deter them but instead find ways around them or even use them as learning opportunities. For instance, consider Sarah, who had been consistent with her exercise regime until she sustained an ankle sprain while hiking. Instead of letting this setback derail her progress entirely, she switched from high-impact exercises like running to low-impact ones like swimming until her ankle healed completely.

Sarah's story is a classic example of how to adapt to challenges. She analysed her situation, devised a solution, and implemented it. A study published in the American Journal of Clinical Nutrition (Klem et al., 1997) highlighted that individuals who maintained their fat loss over time were those who adjusted their dietary intake and physical activity levels based on changes in lifestyle or body weight.

Here are some tips to prepare for unexpected changes:

- Have an alternative workout plan: It could be due to weather conditions or equipment unavailability at the gym.

- Make your diet flexible: If certain foods are not available, know what substitutes you can use without compromising your nutrition goals.

- Work on stress management techniques: Stress might lead to emotional eating, which may affect your progress negatively.

Research reveals that only about one in every five dieters maintain long-term fat loss. This statistic underscores the importance of resilience and mental fortitude during this journey. Obesity and related diseases have been identified as a public health crisis. Energy-dense diets and sedentary lifestyles are the key reasons for obesity. Changing behaviours to reduce disease burden is recognised as the best antidote to the issue of belly fat plaguing us (Wing & Phelan, 2005).

The following steps will guide you through dealing with unexpected challenges:

1. Acknowledge the Situation: Understand that change is inevitable.

2. Analyse: Consider how these changes impact your routine and brainstorm possible solutions.

3. Act: Implement these solutions promptly to minimise any negative effect on your progress.

4. Adjust: Be open-minded enough to adjust if things do not work out as expected initially.

5. Advance: Keep moving forward regardless of setbacks; remember that every step counts, however small it may seem.

Embracing this approach helps build resilience, equipping you better not just for this fitness journey but for life's ups and downs in general. Remember, it is not about how fast you are moving. Push relentlessly in the correct direction, and success is bound to be yours.

Key Takeaways

- Acceptance of possible setbacks lays the foundation for resilience in your fitness journey.

- Adaptability is essential to long-term success.

- Being prepared will help you stay committed even when faced with obstacles.

- Mental strength plays a significant role in overcoming hurdles on your fitness journey.

- Consistently aiming for a lifestyle change for better overall health instead of aiming for weight loss as the end goal will help achieve results faster and more sustainably.

Conclusion

Chapter 34:
Making Peace With Your Body—Self-Love and Acceptance

Throughout this book, we have been on a journey exploring the complex world of belly fat. We have dug deep into why it is so stubbornly attached to our bodies and how it can be an indicator of underlying health issues. We have also dissected various ways to bid it farewell sustainably. But let us halt for a moment and ponder: is not our relentless pursuit to lose belly fat somewhere reflective of our war against our own bodies?

Let us pause here for a second and imagine your body as a faithful companion who has been with you since birth. It has weathered all storms with you, celebrated your victories, cried in your defeats, yet stood by you unwaveringly. Imagine if that loyal friend was constantly criticised or blamed for not being perfect enough. How would they feel? This is what happens when we incessantly focus on losing belly fat or achieving an ideal body image. Our bodies are not just vessels carrying us through life; they are living entities deserving of love and acceptance.

The essence comes from striking the right balance between wanting to improve health (which might involve shedding some pounds) and still loving ourselves during every step of that journey. The key is self-love and acceptance. Self-acceptance does not mean giving up on healthy goals or ignoring potential risks associated with excessive belly fat. Instead, it means acknowledging where we are right now—without judgement—while simultaneously working towards better health outcomes.

In the following words often attributed to the Buddha, "You yourself, as much as anybody in the entire universe, deserve your love and affection." So, treat your body kindly, appreciate its resilience despite all that you have put it through, and cherish its uniqueness.

If we look at this journey from a different perspective—one filled with compassion rather than criticism—we are more likely to stick to healthier habits because they are an act of self-love, not punishment. It is fun to eat nourishing foods and enjoy physical activity when we are doing it out of love for our bodies, not disdain. If you find yourself in a rut or if the problem seems extra bad, seek professional help. A dietician or fitness trainer can guide you through this journey scientifically and healthily. Remember, there is no shame in seeking help. Commonly, people follow crash diets or strenuous exercise regimes, believing they will lose fat quickly. However, these practices can harm your body and are far from sustainable solutions.

Remember that the aim is not an ideal body but consistent progress. Every small step towards a healthier lifestyle counts and is worth celebrating!

Key Takeaways

- Embrace your body as it is right now.
- Aim for better health outcomes rather than just fat loss.
- Treat every step towards a healthier lifestyle as an act of self-love.
- Avoid harmful practices like crash dieting or over-exercising.
- Seek professional help if needed.

Chapter 35:

Maintaining the Momentum—Creating a Lifelong Plan for Health

It does not matter how slowly you go as long as you do not stop. –Confucius

As we cross the finish line of this life-changing journey, it is essential to reflect on everything you have learned so far about belly fat. It can be daunting, yes, but also empowering. You are now equipped with the knowledge needed to make informed decisions about your health and well-being.

Belly fat is not just an aesthetic issue; it is a significant contributor to various health problems such as diabetes, heart disease, and even some types of cancer. Therein lies its danger—not in how it makes us look but in what it signals beneath the surface. Many people are unaware that our bodies store excess energy, such as visceral fat, around vital organs like the liver and pancreas. This is why reducing belly fat is not merely a vanity project—it is a matter of life or death.

Now that you understand this reality, let's talk about maintaining momentum in your fight against belly fat. Studies have shown that losing weight and keeping it off requires more than just temporary diet changes or sporadic exercise routines. The key comes from sustainable lifestyle modifications—small adjustments made over time—that lead to long-lasting results.

Take Maria, for instance; she successfully lost 50 pounds over six months through consistent exercise and healthy eating habits. However, her real success story began after she reached her target weight and managed to maintain her new lifestyle choices without reverting to old patterns.

Analysing Maria's case shows that one size doesn't fit all when it comes to body weight management strategies. She found balance by combining physical activity with mindful eating rather than resorting to extreme diets or punishing workout regimes, proving that there is no 'magic bullet' for fat loss.

A study published in the Journal of Nutrition and Dietetics also supports this notion. It found that people who successfully maintain their fat loss generally adopt a balanced, less restrictive approach to eating combined with regular physical activity (Kruseman & Carrard, 2016).

1. Start by setting realistic goals.

2. Practice mindful eating; learn to eat when you are hungry and stop when you are full.

3. Stay active and incorporate movement into your daily routine.

1. Tracking your progress and acknowledging small victories along the way will help you feel motivated.

Surprisingly, one-third of American adults are obese, according to CDC data from 2015–2018 (*Physical Activity Basics*, 2019). That is a staggering statistic—one that underscores the importance of understanding body fat management strategies, especially as it pertains to belly fat.

As you move forward with the effort you put in towards better health, remember these action steps:

1. Prioritise consistency over intensity in both diet and exercise.

2. Avoid short-term diet fads; instead, focus on developing healthy eating habits that can be maintained in the long run.

3. Set achievable fitness goals, like walking for half an hour every day, rather than aiming for high-intensity workouts right away.

4. Monitor your progress regularly, but do not obsess over numbers on scales; they are just tools, not determinants of success or failure.

5. Finally, seek support if necessary, whether from healthcare professionals or loved ones, because nobody should have to embark on this journey alone.

If taken seriously, these steps can help you make sense of everything we have discussed in this book about belly fat—and, more importantly, help you live a healthier life free from the dangers of excess belly fat. Belly fat is a widespread issue, and millions of lives are lost worldwide. However, since visceral fat is metabolically active, a healthy routine and consistent efforts can help banish it and prevent it from appearing again. Consistency is the keyword, and aim for progress, not perfection!

Key Takeaways

- Belly fat is more than an aesthetic issue; it significantly contributes to various health problems.

- Sustainable lifestyle modifications are the key to long-lasting fat loss results.

- There is no 'magic bullet' for weight loss—balance is key.

- The prevalence of obesity highlights the need for sustainable body fat management strategies.

Food Portions: A Quick Guide

Diet and eating right play a huge role in beating that belly bulge. However, counting the macros and calories of each item of food you put in your body can be daunting. It can make us obsess over food and cause stress, which is not doing you any good in the fight against the burgeoning waistline. This is where a simple guide to portion sizes can standardise your meals and make it easy to track the nutrients available to your body.

First of all, it is very important to understand that each food group serves your body in different ways. Eliminating any one food group is neither desirable nor sustainable in the long run. The key to eating right is eating all food groups in moderation! Protein is required for healthy muscle function. It is responsible for the repair of wear and tear and is also responsible for the building and strengthening of skeletal muscles.

As discussed earlier, more muscle mass increases our resting metabolic rate, which means that you continue burning energy and excess fat long after you are done with your workouts! Carbohydrates and fats provide the energy required for your body to carry out its day-to-day functions. It helps keep the body well-hydrated and working optimally. Finally, fruits and vegetables provide water-soluble fibre essential for gut health, along with a host of other vitamins and minerals that the body needs for optimal health!

A simple way to incorporate all the essential components while also ensuring a healthy calorific intake is to use your palm to measure your food! Yes, you heard it right. Keep aside those fancy weighing scales and apps. You do not need precision when starting a healthy diet. What counts is consistency, and hence, a simple way to track food is essential when it comes to a sustainable diet.

Proteins

Proteins can be broadly classified as proteins from meat sources and proteins from non-meat sources. For optimal long-term health, try to incorporate both sources of protein in each of your three meals a day! **One serving of meat protein** must be approximately the **size of your clenched fist**. Make sure to include **another serving of non-meat protein the size of your clenched fist**. Let us now look into the most commonly consumed protein sources.

Meat protein sources may include:

- Steamed/boiled fish

- Grilled/Curried chicken

Try to avoid processed meats, as they tend to have a lot of chemical additives that work as both preservatives and condiments. It is also high in sodium from the curing process. Processed meats include sausages, ham, deli meats, and bacon. Fish and chicken are lean sources of protein with relatively fewer saturated fats than red meats.

Non-meat sources of protein include:

- Broccoli

- Soy Milk

- Eggs

- Mushrooms

- Tofu

Plant-based foods can also be sources of antioxidants, minerals, and vitamins that can boost overall health!

Carbohydrates

Carbohydrates are the energy powerhouse. It acts as fuel for the body to perform its day-to-day tasks, from breathing and involuntary muscle movements to the high-impact training you do at the gym. Hence, consuming carbohydrates and not completely cutting them out of your diet is important.

Try to include carbohydrates that have a low glycaemic index (that is, the rate at which the sugars are released into your blood). A low glycaemic index ensures that you stay satiated for longer and also prevents blood sugar spikes.

Also, stay away from highly processed foods and grains. Processed and refined sugars are also known to create spikes in blood sugar and hamper digestion and metabolism. A simple way to pick your carbohydrates would be to avoid packaged ready-to-eat products and opt for traditional and less processed food.

A serving of carbohydrates should ideally fit your cupped palm. The body breaks down the complex carbohydrates and starches into glucose for use in the body.

Healthy sources of carbohydrates may include:

- Brown rice

- Whole wheat bread, naan, or roti

- Oats

Fruits and Vegetables

As kids, we have always been instructed to eat our veggies to be taller, stronger, cleverer, and whatnot! There is a good reason for this! Fruits and vegetables are loaded with nutrients and minerals that keep the body functioning as it should. Elements vital for body functioning, like potassium, calcium, magnesium, and iron, are obtained from fruits and vegetables. They also contain water-soluble fibres essential for good gut health, digestion, and waste elimination. They are highly beneficial for brain, skin, and hair health!!

Always try to add a variety of fruits and vegetables of different colours to your diet. The compounds that give the various veggies their hues are also highly nutritious for the body. For example., thylakoids in spinach, curcumin in turmeric, carotenoids in carrots, and anthocyanins in blueberries! They are known to be potent antioxidants capable of fighting inflammation and promoting overall health. Make sure to consume fruits high in sugar in moderation, especially if you aim to monitor blood glucose. For fruits, a **handful of berries or a fist size fruit**. Minimally, **cooked veggies should cover one palm** (including your fingers!), **double up to 2 palms if veggies are raw** like a salad.

Fruits and vegetables you could consider including in your diet:

- Green leafy vegetables are the only food you could go to town with!

- Tomato

- Carrots and beets

- Apples, Oranges and Kiwis

Consider the following meal plan for a week. You could use this as a reference point and build your meals around it! I lived in Singapore half my life and Australia for the other half - below meal plan reflects my food choices. Feel free to link up with me if you would like me to help design a meal plan for you!

Monday

Breakfast: Chapati, lentil dal, chicken tikka and apple

Lunch: Steamed white rice, Assam steamed fish, stir-fried chinese spinach with garlic and chili and guava

Dinner: Steamed white rice, minced chicken, steamed tofu and stir-fried cabbage

Tuesday

Breakfast: Oatmeal muffins, low-fat milk, boiled egg, strawberry and blueberries

Lunch: Steamed brown rice, stir-fried broccoli and carrot, steamed fish and guava

Dinner: Baked potatoes, grilled mushroom, grilled chicken thighs, lettuce and tomatoes

Wednesday

Breakfast: Tuna sandwich with vegetables, soya milk and an orange

Lunch: Steamed white rice, steamed egg, steamed chicken and stir-fried green vegetables

Dinner: Quinoa, boiled broccoli, grilled salmon, lettuce and tomato balsamic vinaigrette salad

Thursday

Breakfast: Mee Hoon soup, bean sprouts, sliced chicken breast and apple

Lunch: Steamed white rice, pan-fried cod with soy sauce, bean curd with bean sprouts, blanched cai xin and apple

Dinner: Shio Ramen, onsen egg, sliced pork, leeks and beanshoots, and nashi pear

Friday

Breakfast: Oatmeal with low-fat milk, boiled eggs, kiwi and strawberries

Lunch: Wanton mee, low sugar soy milk, BBQ chicken breast and green vegetables

Dinner: Spaghetti, mushroom sauté, minced chicken, and kiwi

Saturday

Breakfast: Multi-grain biscuits, low-fat milk, scrambled eggs and papaya

Lunch: Steamed white rice, steamed chicken, boiled bean sprouts, kimchi greens and orange

Dinner: Steamed white rice, boiled egg, fish curry with okra, and starfruit

Sunday

Breakfast: Chicken salad with lettuce, cherry tomato and corn and boiled egg

Lunch: Roasted chicken whole wheat wrap, hummus and orange

Dinner: Sweet potato, grilled fish, pan-roasted mixed vegetables

As discussed earlier, sometimes, food alone can be inadequate in providing all the nutrients required for the body to function in a healthy manner. Vitamin B12 is one such nutrient which may be difficult to obtain, especially from a fully plant-based diet. Other elements, too, could be deficient or completely lacking when depending on food for all vitamins and minerals.

Other minerals include iron, iodine, potassium, magnesium, and vitamin A. It is always a good idea to get a vitamin profile test done. Well-formulated supplements can correct deficiencies. Make sure to opt for a trusted and science-backed brand when choosing supplements. Look for supplements that have omega fats and antioxidant properties.

Glossary

Adrenaline: A hormone produced by the adrenal gland that helps you react to stress, often characterised as a "fight or flight response."

Alpha receptor: Alpha receptors are proteins that cause muscle contraction or constriction by attaching themselves to signalling molecules.

Anthocyanins: Anthocyanins are a type of flavonoid commonly found in red, purple, or blue fruits and vegetables. Types of berries, apples, black grapes, plums, and purple cabbage are rich in anthocyanins.

Antioxidants: Substances either occurring in nature or manufactured in a laboratory that prevent or slow certain types of oxidative cell damage. Antioxidants are naturally found in many foods, including certain fruits and vegetables. They are also available as nutritional supplements.

Beiging: The process of white adipose tissue (WAT) gaining the properties of brown adipose tissue (BAT) over time.

Beta receptor: Beta receptors are proteins that cause muscle relaxation and dilation by binding themselves to signalling molecules.

Brown adipose tissue (BAT): A type of fat or adipose tissue with a high concentration of mitochondria, specialised in energy expenditure and thermogenesis.

Cortisol: A steroid hormone that is produced by your two adrenal glands, located on top of each kidney. The hormone is released into the bloodstream in a situation of high stress.

Cytokines: Tiny proteins that are important for the growth and activity of other immune system cells and blood cells. It affects cells that help the body's immune and inflammation responses.

Endocrine system: A network of glands and organs producing and utilising hormones to manage and coordinate the body's metabolic functions, energy level, reproduction, growth and development, repair wear and tear, and mood.

Flavonoid: Phytochemical compounds present in many plants, fruits, vegetables, and leaves that are found to be chemically crucial for maintaining a healthy life.

Free radicals: Free radicals are high-energy atoms that can cause oxidative damage to cells, causing various types of illnesses and aging.

High-Density Lipoprotein (HDL): HDL transports cholesterol from the peripheral tissues to the liver and has anti-inflammatory properties, reducing plaque and its associated inflammation.

High-Intensity Interval Training (HIIT): A type of physical training exercise that involves repeated rounds that mix several minutes of high-intensity motion to increase the heart rate to at least 80% of the maximum rate, followed by short periods of rest or lower-intensity movements.

Homeostasis: A state of equilibrium among all the body systems, like the circulatory, nervous, digestive, and reproductive, needed for the body to survive and function correctly.

Insulin resistance: Insulin resistance is a condition when cells in your muscles, fat, and liver do not respond well to insulin and cannot easily take up glucose from your blood.

Isometric exercise: An exercise involving the static steady-state hold of multiple muscle groups without any perceptible movement in the body.

Lean Protein: Lean protein is a food that is high in protein but low in saturated fat.

Low-Density Lipoprotein (LDL): LDL leads to a buildup of cholesterol, a waxy substance found in all the cells in your body, and plaque in arteries.

Meditation: Meditation is a practice involving mental and physical techniques to improve brain health and overall well-being.

Metabolic syndrome: Metabolic syndrome is a group of multiple conditions that can lead to coronary disease, diabetes, kidney problems, and other health problems. The five conditions include high blood glucose, low levels of HDL ("good") cholesterol, high levels of LDL ("bad") cholesterol, a large waist circumference, and high blood pressure.

Metabolism: The process by which the body's cells change food into energy to perform physical and mental activities like moving, thinking, and growing.

Mindfulness: A type of meditation practice in which you are acutely aware of what you are experiencing and feeling in the moment, without explanation or judgment.

Monounsaturated fats: The type of fats found in plant foods, such as nuts, avocados, and vegetable oils, that have healthy benefits for the functioning of the heart.

Neurotransmitters: Neurotransmitters are molecules that transmit chemical signals from one nerve cell to the next target cell. These signals help produce responses in muscles and glands.

Nicotine: A naturally occurring chemical in tobacco that is used as a recreational stimulant. It is addictive and speeds up the transmission of messages in your nerve cells.

Subcutaneous fat: The layer of fat tissue between the skin and muscles.

Visceral fat: Fat accumulated within the abdominal wall and around internal organs such as the intestines and kidneys.

Omega-3 fatty acids: Found in foods, such as fish and chia seeds, and nutritional supplements, like cod liver oil, and have many benefits for your heart, circulatory system, lungs, nervous system, and endocrinological system.

Omentum: A fold of thin tissue that lines the abdomen surrounding the stomach and other organs in the abdomen.

Pilates: A low-impact, controlled exercise comprising slow and deliberate movements to improve balance, core strength, agility, and even the state of mind.

Resistance training: A form of exercise to increase strength and endurance while performing aerobic activities and increase the volume of skeletal muscle. It involves the use of muscle groups against gravity's effect on weights or your own body weight.

Serotonin: A produced by the intestines and brain. It helps transmit signals between cells of the nervous system, affecting mood, emotional regulation, and digestion.

Soluble Fibre: Fibre found in foods such as oat bran, nuts, seeds, beans, lentils, and some fruits and vegetables that dissolve in water.

Thylakoid: Sacs found in the membrane of the chloroplasts of a plant cell, containing chlorophyll that absorbs light for use in photosynthesis and other light-dependent processes.

Triglyceride: The most common type of fat or lipid in the human body that circulates in the blood. It is responsible for LDL or bad cholesterol.

White adipose tissue (WAT): White adipose tissue is comprised of fat cells specialised for energy storage.

Yoga: Yoga is a form of low- to moderate-intensity exercise that originated in ancient India. It integrates the mind, body, and the spiritual and is proven to build strength and flexibility.

References

Abdominal fat and what to do about it. (2019, June 25). Harvard Health. https://www.health.harvard.edu/staying-healthy/abdominal-fat-and-what-to-do-about-it

American Academy of Neurology. (2019, January 9). Excessive body fat around the middle linked to smaller brain size, study finds. *ScienceDaily.* www.sciencedaily.com/releases/2019/01/190109164233.htm

American heart association recommendations for physical activity in adults and kids. (2018, April 18). American Heart Association. https://www.heart.org/en/healthy-living/fitness/fitness-basics/aha-recs-for-physical-activity-in-adults

Beck, M. (n.d.). *Martha Beck quotes.* BrainyQuote. https://www.brainyquote.com/quotes/martha_beck_282605

Belly fat in women: Get rid of it — for good! (2023, June 28). Mayo Clinic. https://www.mayoclinic.org/healthy-lifestyle/womens-health/in-depth/belly-fat/art-20045809

Bertoia, M. L., Rimm, E. B., Mukamal, K. J., Hu, F. B., Willett, W. C., & Cassidy, A. (2016). Dietary flavonoid intake and weight maintenance: three prospective cohorts of 124 086 US men and women followed for up to 24 years. *BMJ, 352*(17), 17. https://doi.org/10.1136/bmj.i17

Bhardwaj, R. L., Parashar, A., Parewa, H. P., & Vyas, L. (2024). An alarming decline in the nutritional quality of foods: The biggest challenge for future generations' health. *Foods, 13*(6), 877. https://doi.org/10.3390/foods13060877

Billings, J. (n.d.). *Josh Billings quotes.* A-Z Quotes. https://www.azquotes.com/author/1398-Josh_Billings

Bilodeau, K. (2018, July 26). Belly fat linked with higher heart disease risk. *Harvard Health Blog.* https://www.health.harvard.edu/blog/belly-fat-linked-with-higher-heart-disease-risk-2018072614354

Blessing, W., Mohammed, M., & Ootsuka, Y. (2012). Heating and eating: Brown adipose tissue thermogenesis precedes food ingestion as part of the ultradian basic rest–activity cycle in rats. *Physiology & Behavior*, *105*(4), 966–974. https://doi.org/10.1016/j.physbeh.2011.11.009

Brown, T., Avenell, A., Edmunds, L. D., Moore, H., Whittaker, V., Avery, L., & Summerbell, C. (2009). Systematic review of long-term lifestyle interventions to prevent weight gain and morbidity in adults. *Obesity reviews*, *10*(6), 627–638. https://doi.org/10.1111/j.1467-789x.2009.00641.x

Buddha. (n.d). *Buddha quotes.* Brainy Quote. https://www.brainyquote.com/quotes/buddha_132910

Callahan, A., PhD, Leonard, H., MEd, RDN, Powell, T., MS, & RDN. (2020, October 14). *Nutrition in Older Adults.* Openoregon.pressbooks.pub. https://openoregon.pressbooks.pub/nutritionscience/chapter/11f-older-adults/

Canfield, J. (n.d). Jack Canfield quotes. Goodreads. https://www.goodreads.com/author/quotes/35476.Jack_Canfield

Carrasquilla, G. D., García-Ureña, M., Romero-Lado, M. J., & Kilpeläinen, T. O. (2024). Estimating causality between smoking and abdominal obesity by Mendelian randomization. *Addiction*. https://doi.org/10.1111/add.16454

Cassidy, A., Mukamal, K. J., Liu, L., Franz, M., Eliassen, A. H., & Rimm, E. B. (2013). High anthocyanin intake is associated with a reduced risk of myocardial infarction in young and middle-aged women. *Circulation*, *127*(2), 188–196. https://doi.org/10.1161/circulationaha.112.122408

Cerhan, J. R., Moore, S. C., Jacobs, E. J., Kitahara, C. M., Rosenberg, P. S., Adami, H.-O., Ebbert, J. O., English, D. R., Gapstur, S. M., Giles, G. G., Horn-Ross, P. L., Park, Y., Patel, A. V., Robien, K., Weiderpass, E., Willett, W. C., Wolk, A., Zeleniuch-Jacquotte, A., Hartge, P., & Bernstein, L. (2014). A pooled analysis of waist circumference and mortality in 650,000 adults. *Mayo Clinic proceedings*, *89*(3), 335–345. https://doi.org/10.1016/j.mayocp.2013.11.011

Chatkin, R., Chatkin, J. M., Spanemberg, L., Casagrande, D., Wagner, M., & Mottin, C. (2015). Smoking is associated with more abdominal fat in morbidly obese patients. *PLOS ONE*, *10*(5), e0126146. https://doi.org/10.1371/journal.pone.0126146

Cherpak, C. E. (2019). Mindful eating: a review of how the stress-digestion-mindfulness triad may modulate and improve gastrointestinal and digestive function. *Integrative medicine (Encinitas, Calif.)*, *18*(4), 48–53. https://europepmc.org/article/med/32549835

Collins, S. (2023, December 19). *The truth about belly fat*. WebMD. https://www.webmd.com/diet/features/the-truth-about-belly-fat

Couet, C., Delarue, J., Ritz, P., Antoine, J. M., & Lamisse, F. (1997). Effect of dietary fish oil on body fat mass and basal fat oxidation in healthy adults. *International journal of obesity and related metabolic disorders: journal of the international association for the study of obesity*, *21*(8), 637–643. https://doi.org/10.1038/sj.ijo.0800451

Cohen, A. P. (n.d.). *Peter A. Cohen quotes*. https://proverbhunter.com/quote/there-is-no-one-giant-step-that-does-it-its-a-lot-of-little-steps/

Cramer, H., Thoms, M. S., Anheyer, D., Lauche, R., & Dobos, G. (2016). Yoga in Women With Abdominal Obesity. *Deutsches Aerzteblatt Online*, *113*(39). https://doi.org/10.3238/arztebl.2016.0645

Confucius. (n.d.). Confucius quotes. Brainy Quote. https://www.brainyquote.com/quotes/confucius_140908

Dempsey, P. C., Larsen, R. N., Sethi, P., Sacre, J. W., Straznicky, N. E., Cohen, N. D., Cerin, E., Lambert, G. W., Owen, N., Kingwell, B. A., & Dunstan, D. W. (2016). Benefits for type 2 diabetes of interrupting prolonged sitting with brief bouts of light walking or simple resistance activities. *Diabetes Care, 39*(6), 964–972. https://doi.org/10.2337/dc15-2336

Drehmer, M., Suzi Alves Camey, Maria Angélica Nunes, Bruce Bartholow Duncan, Lacerda, M., Andréia Poyastro Pinheiro, & María Inês Schmidt. (2012). Fibre intake and evolution of BMI: from pre-pregnancy to postpartum. *Public health nutrition, 16*(8), 1403–1413. https://doi.org/10.1017/s1368980012003849

Drucker, P. (n.d.). *Peter Drucker quotes*. BrainyQuotes. https://www.brainyquote.com/quotes/peter_drucker_131600

Duhigg, C. (n.d.). *Charles Duhigg quote*. Goodreads. https://www.goodreads.com/author/quotes/5201530.Charles_Duhigg

Dutcher, J. M. (2022). Brain reward circuits promote stress resilience and health: implications for reward-based interventions. *Current directions in psychological science, 32*(1), 096372142211217. https://doi.org/10.1177/09637214221121770

Dyett, L. (2022, April 28). Martha Stewart welcomes you to generation ageless. *The New York Times*. https://www.nytimes.com/2022/04/28/style/martha-stewart-tiktok.html

Edison, T. A. (n.d.). *Thomas A. Edison quotes*. Goodreads. https://www.goodreads.com/quotes/13639-the-doctor-of-the-future-will-give-no-medication-but

Einstein, T. A. (n.d.). *Albert Einstien quotes*. Goodreads. https://www.goodreads.com/quotes/29213-life-is-like-riding-a-bicycle-to-keep-your-balance

Eliot, G. (n.d.). *George Eliot quotes*. Brainy Quote. https://www.brainyquote.com/quotes/george_eliot_161679

Frankel, B. (n.d.). Bethenny Frankel quotes. Brainy Quote. https://www.brainyquote.com/quotes/bethenny_frankel_482602

Frayling, T. M., Timpson, N. J., Weedon, M. N., Zeggini, E., Freathy, R. M., Lindgren, C. M., Perry, J. R. B., Elliott, K. S., Lango, H., Rayner, N. W., Shields, B., Harries, L. W., Barrett, J. C., Ellard, S., Groves, C. J., Knight, B., Patch, A.-M. ., Ness, A. R., Ebrahim, S., & Lawlor, D. A. (2007). A Common variant in the FTO gene is associated with body mass index and predisposes to childhood and adult obesity. *Science*, *316*(5826), 889–894. https://doi.org/10.1126/science.1141634

Fuller, T. (n.d.). *Thomas Fuller quotes*. BrainyQuote. https://www.brainyquote.com/quotes/thomas_fuller_380713

Godsey, J. (2013). The role of mindfulness based interventions in the treatment of obesity and eating disorders: An integrative review. *Complementary therapies in Medicine*, *21*(4), 430-439. https://doi.org/10.1016/j.ctim.2013.06.003

Hajek, T. (2021, August 12). Obesity is a risk factor for brain-structure changes in schizophrenia and bipolar disorder, 2 studies show. *Brain & Behavior Research Foundation*. https://bbrfoundation.org/content/obesity-risk-factor-brain-structure-changes-schizophrenia-and-bipolar-disorder-2-studies

Hanlon, E. C., Tasali, E., Leproult, R., Stuhr, K. L., Doncheck, E., de Wit, H., Hillard, C. J., & Van Cauter, E. (2016). Sleep restriction enhances the daily rhythm of circulating levels of endocannabinoid 2-arachidonoylglycerol. *Sleep*, *39*(3), 653–664. https://doi.org/10.5665/sleep.5546

Henson, J., Edwardson, C. L., Morgan, B., Horsfield, M. A., Khunti, K., Davies, M. J., & Yates, T. (2017). Sedentary time and mri-derived measures of adiposity in active versus inactive individuals. *Obesity*, *26*(1), 29–36. https://doi.org/10.1002/oby.22034

Hippocrates. (n.d.). *Hippocrates quotes*. Goodreads. https://www.goodreads.com/quotes/tag/food

Huffington, A. (n.d.). *Arianna Huffington quotes*. A-Z Quotes. https://www.azquotes.com/quote/638033

Hurt, R. T., Kulisek, C., Buchanan, L. A., & McClave, S. A. (2010). The obesity epidemic: challenges, health initiatives, and implications for gastroenterologists. Gastroenterology & Hepatology, 6(12), 780–792. https://www.ncbi.nlm.nih.gov/pmc/articles/PMC3033553/

Hyman, M. (n.d.). *Mark Hyman quotes.* Total Wellness. https://info.totalwellnesshealth.com/blog/quotes-on-wellness-and-health

Indicator metadata registry details. (n.d.). World Health Organization. https://www.who.int/data/gho/indicator-metadata-registry/imr-details/3416

Item, F., & Konrad, D. (2012). Visceral fat and metabolic inflammation: the portal theory revisited. *Obesity reviews, 13,* 30–39. https://doi.org/10.1111/j.1467-789x.2012.01035.x

Ivey, K. L., Jensen, M. K., Hodgson, J. M., Eliassen, A. H., Cassidy, A., & Rimm, E. B. (2017). Association of flavonoid-rich foods and flavonoids with risk of all-cause mortality. *British journal of nutrition, 117*(10), 1470–1477. https://doi.org/10.1017/S0007114517001325

James, P. T., Leach, R., Kalamara, E., & Shayeghi, M. (2001). The Worldwide Obesity Epidemic. *Obesity Research, 9*(S11), 228S233S. https://doi.org/10.1038/oby.2001.123

Jastreboff, A. M., Sinha, R., Lacadie, C., Small, D. M., Sherwin, R. S., & Potenza, M. N. (2013). Neural correlates of stress- and food cue-induced food craving in obesity: association with insulin levels. *Diabetes care, 36*(2), 394–402. https://doi.org/10.2337/dc12-1112

Jordan, M. (n.d.). *Michael Jordan quotes.* Brainy Quote. https://www.brainyquote.com/quotes/michael_jordan_165967

Joyner-Kersee. J. (n.d.). Jackie Joyner-Kersee quotes. Brainy Quotes. https://www.brainyquote.com/quotes/jackie_joynerkersee_126146

Judd, N. (n.d). Naomi Judd quotes. BrainyQuote. https://www.brainyquote.com/quotes/naomi_judd_170356

Klem, M. L., Wing, R. R., McGuire, M. T., Seagle, H. M., & Hill, J. O. (1997). A descriptive study of individuals successful at long-term maintenance of substantial weight loss. *The American journal of clinical nutrition*, *66*(2), 239–246. https://doi.org/10.1093/ajcn/66.2.239

Koban, L., Wager, T. D., & Kober, H. (2022). A neuromarker for drug and food craving distinguishes drug users from non-users. *Nature Neuroscience*, *26*, 316–325. https://doi.org/10.1038/s41593-022-01228-w

Kristeller, J. L., & Wolever, R. Q. (2010). Mindfulness-based eating awareness training for treating binge eating disorder: the conceptual foundation. *Eating disorders*, *19*(1), 49–61. https://doi.org/10.1080/10640266.2011.533605

Kruseman, M., & Carrard, I. (2016). Physical activity and weight loss maintenance: practice and perceptions. *Journal of the academy of nutrition and dietetics*, *116*(9), A89. https://doi.org/10.1016/j.jand.2016.06.322

Lafontan, M., & Berlan, M. (1993). Fat cell adrenergic receptors and the control of white and brown fat cell function. *Journal of lipid research*, *34*(7), 1057–1091. https://pubmed.ncbi.nlm.nih.gov/8371057/

Lan, N., Lu, Y., Zhang, Y., Pu, S., Xi, H., Nie, X., Liu, J., & Yuan, W. (2020). FTO – A common genetic basis for obesity and cancer. *Frontiers in genetics*, *11*. https://doi.org/10.3389/fgene.2020.559138

Li, D., Lee, J., Li, Y., & Li, C. (2011). Natural products and body weight control. *North American journal of medical sciences*, *3*(1), 13. https://doi.org/10.4297/najms.2011.313

LeWine, H. E. (2012, August 8). *Diabetes can strike—hard—even when weight is normal.* Harvard Health. https://www.health.harvard.edu/blog/diabetes-can-strike-hard-even-when-weight-is-normal-201208085121

Li, Y., Pan, A., Wang, D. D., Liu, X., Dhana, K., Franco, O. H., Kaptoge, S., Di Angelantonio, E., Stampfer, M., Willett, W. C., & Hu, F. B. (2018). Impact of healthy lifestyle factors on life expectancies in the US population. *Circulation, 138*(4), 345–355. https://doi.org/10.1161/circulationaha.117.032047

Liu, F., Flatt, S., Nichols, J., Pakiz, B., Barkai, H., Wing, D., Heath, D., & Rock, C. (2017). Factors associated with visceral fat loss in response to a multifaceted weight loss intervention. *Journal of obesity & weight loss therapy, 7*(4). https://doi.org/10.4172/2165-7904.1000346

Lockett, Eleesha (2023, March 22). *How does alcohol affect weight loss?* Healthline; Healthline Media. https://www.healthline.com/health/alcohol-and-weight-loss

Loos, R. J. F., & Yeo, G. S. H. (2013). The bigger picture of FTO—the first GWAS-identified obesity gene. *Nature reviews Endocrinology, 10*(1), 51–61. https://doi.org/10.1038/nrendo.2013.227

Lopes, H. F., Corrêa-Giannella, M. L., Consolim-Colombo, F. M., & Egan, B. M. (2016). Visceral adiposity syndrome. *Diabetology & metabolic syndrome, 8*(1). https://doi.org/10.1186/s13098-016-0156-2

Maté, G. (n.d.). *Gabor Maté quotes*. Goodreads. https://www.goodreads.com/quotes/tag/addiction?page=1

Metabolic syndrome: causes and risk factors. (2022, May 18). National Heart, Lung, and Blood Institute. https://www.nhlbi.nih.gov/health/metabolic-syndrome/causes

Miller, D. (n.d.). *Dan Miller Quotes*. Goodreads. https://www.goodreads.com/quotes/2232590-the-secret-of-change-is-to-focus-all-your-energy

Miller, S. (2020, February 27). The diet industrial complex got me, and it will never let me go. *New York Times*. https://www.nytimes.com/2020/02/26/style/body-positive-movement.html

Mindful eating. (2011, February). Harvard Health. https://www.health.harvard.edu/staying-healthy/mindful-eating

More belly weight increases danger of heart disease even if BMI does not indicate obesity. (2021, April). American Heart Association. https://newsroom.heart.org/news/more-belly-weight-increases-danger-of-heart-disease-even-if-bmi-does-not-indicate-obesity

Mozaffarian, D., & Wu, J. H. Y. (2018). Flavonoids, dairy foods, and cardiovascular and metabolic health. *Circulation research*, *122*(2), 369–384. https://doi.org/10.1161/circresaha.117.309008

Mykkänen, O. T., Huotari, A., Herzig, K.-H., Dunlop, T. W., Mykkänen, H., & Kirjavainen, P. V. (2014). Wild blueberries (vaccinium myrtillus) alleviate inflammation and hypertension associated with developing obesity in mice fed with a high-fat diet. *PLoS ONE*, *9*(12), e114790. https://doi.org/10.1371/journal.pone.0114790

Obesity and overweight. (2024, March 1). World Health Organization. https://www.who.int/news-room/fact-sheets/detail/obesity-and-overweight

Obesity-related cardiovascular disease deaths tripled between 1999 and 2020. (2023, September 6). American Heart Association. https://newsroom.heart.org/news/obesity-related-cardiovascular-disease-deaths-tripled-between-1999-and-2020

Okunogbe, A., Nugent, R., Spencer, G., Powis, J., Ralston, J., & Wilding, J. (2022). Economic impacts of overweight and obesity: current and future estimates for 161 countries. *BMJ global health*, *7*(9). https://doi.org/10.1136/bmjgh-2022-009773

Oliveira, B. F., Chang, C. R., Oetsch, K., Falkenhain, K., Crampton, K., Stork, M., Hoonjan, M., Elliott, T., Francois, M. E., & Little, J. P. (2023). Impact of a Low-Carbohydrate Compared with Low-Fat Breakfast on Blood Glucose Control in Type 2 Diabetes: A Randomized Trial. *The American journal of clinical nutrition*, *118*(1), 209-217. https://doi.org/10.1016/j.ajcnut.2023.04.032

O'Toole, M. L., Sawicki, M. A., & Artal, R. (2003). Structured diet and physical activity prevent postpartum weight retention. *Journal of women's health*, *12*(10), 991–998. https://doi.org/10.1089/154099903322643910

Physical activity basics. (2019). Centers for Disease Control and Prevention. https://www.cdc.gov/physicalactivity/basics/index.htm

Pollan, M. (n.d.). *Michael Pollan quotes*. Goodreads. https://www.goodreads.com/quotes/18508-eat-food-not-too-much-mostly-plants

Prevalence of overweight, obesity, and extreme obesity among adults aged 20 and over: United States, 1960–1962 through 2013–2014. (2019). CDC. https://www.cdc.gov/nchs/data/hestat/obesity_adult_15_16/obesity_adult_15_16.htm

Quaglia, S. (2021, August 18). *"Deep fat" study reveals a surprising brain-immune system connection*. Inverse. https://www.inverse.com/mind-body/visceral-fat-study

Rebello, C. J., Chu, J., Beyl, R., Edwall, D., Erlanson-Albertsson, C., & Greenway, F. L. (2015). Acute effects of a spinach extract rich in thylakoids on satiety: A randomized controlled crossover trial. *Journal of the American college of nutrition, 34*(6), 470–477. https://doi.org/10.1080/07315724.2014.1003999

Robert N. Butler: Pioneer in study of aging. (2022, September 26). Columbia University Irving Medical Center. https://www.cuimc.columbia.edu/news/robert-n-butler-pioneer-study-aging

RodrÃguez-MartÃn, B. C., & Meule, A. (2015). Food craving: new contributions on its assessment, moderators, and consequences. *Frontiers in Psychology, 6*. https://doi.org/10.3389/fpsyg.2015.00021

Rohn, J. (n.d.). *Jim Rohn quotes*. Goodreads. https://www.goodreads.com/quotes/561636-your-life-does-not-get-better-by-chance-it-gets

Sandoval, V., Sanz-Lamora, H., Arias, G., Marrero, P. F., Haro, D., & Relat, J. (2020). Metabolic impact of flavonoids consumption in obesity: from central to peripheral. *Nutrients, 12*(8), 2393. https://doi.org/10.3390/nu12082393

Shuster, A., Patlas, M., Pinthus, J. H., & Mourtzakis, M. (2012). The clinical importance of visceral adiposity: a critical review of methods for visceral adipose tissue analysis. *The British journal of radiology, 85*(1009), 1–10. https://doi.org/10.1259/bjr/38447238

Sonko, B., Prentice, A., Murgatroyd, P., Goldberg, G., Van de Ven, M., & Coward, W. (1994). Effect of alcohol on postmeal fat storage. *The American Journal of Clinical Nutrition, 59*(3), 619-625. https://doi.org/10.1093/ajcn/59.3.619

Speliotes, E. K., Willer, C. J., Berndt, S. I., Monda, K. L., Thorleifsson, G., Jackson, A. U., Allen, H. L., Lindgren, C. M., Luan, J., Mägi, R., Randall, J. C., Vedantam, S., Winkler, T. W., Qi, L., Workalemahu, T., Heid, I. M., Steinthorsdottir, V., Stringham, H. M., Weedon, M. N., & Wheeler, E. (2010). Association analyses of 249,796 individuals reveal 18 new loci associated with body mass index. *Nature genetics, 42*(11), 937–948. https://doi.org/10.1038/ng.686

Sumithran, P., Prendergast, L. A., Delbridge, E., Purcell, K., Shulkes, A., Kriketos, A., & Proietto, J. (2011). Long-term persistence of hormonal adaptations to weight loss. *New England journal of medicine, 365*(17), 1597–1604. https://doi.org/10.1056/nejmoa1105816

Sun, C., Kovacs, P., & Guiu-Jurado, E. (2021). Genetics of body fat distribution: comparative analyses in populations with European, Asian and African ancestries. *Genes, 12*(6), 841. https://doi.org/10.3390/genes12060841

Taking aim at belly fat. (2024, March 26). Harvard Health. https://www.health.harvard.edu/staying-healthy/taking-aim-at-belly-fat

The stress-diet connection. (2020, July 22). Tufts Health & Nutrition Letter. https://www.nutritionletter.tufts.edu/healthy-eating/the-stress-diet-connection/

Thyagarajan, B. & Foster, M. (2017). Beiging of white adipose tissue as a therapeutic strategy for weight loss in humans. *Hormone molecular biology and clinical investigation, 31*(2), 20170016. https://doi.org/10.1515/hmbci-2017-0016

Tobias, D. K., & Hu, F. B. (2018). The association between BMI and mortality: implications for obesity prevention. *The Lancet diabetes & endocrinology, 6*(12), 916–917. https://doi.org/10.1016/s2213-8587(18)30309-7

Tracy, B. (n.d.). *Brian Tracy quotes.* Goodreads. https://www.goodreads.com/quotes/23014-the-ability-to-discipline-yourself-to-delay-gratification-in-the

Traversy, G., & Chaput, J.-P. (2018). Alcohol consumption and obesity: an update. *Current Obesity Reports, 4*(1), 122–130. https://doi.org/10.1007/s13679-014-0129-4

Trinei, M., Carpi, A., Menabo', R., Storto, M., Fornari, M., Marinelli, A., Minardi, S., Riboni, M., Casciaro, F., DiLisa, F., Petroni, K., Tonelli, C., & Giorgio, M. (2022). Dietary intake of cyanidin-3-glucoside induces a long-lasting cardioprotection from ischemia/reperfusion injury by altering the microbiota. *The journal of nutritional biochemistry, 101,* 108921. https://doi.org/10.1016/j.jnutbio.2021.108921

Tsuda, T., Horio, F., Uchida, K., Aoki, H., & Osawa, T. (2003). Dietary cyanidin 3-o-β-d-glucoside-rich purple corn color prevents obesity and ameliorates hyperglycemia in mice. *The journal of nutrition, 133*(7), 2125–2130. https://doi.org/10.1093/jn/133.7.2125

Underferth, D. (2017). *How does obesity cause cancer?* MD Anderson Cancer Center. https://www.mdanderson.org/publications/focused-on-health/how-does-obesity-cause-cancer.h27Z1591413.html

van Egmond, L. T., Meth, E. M. S., Engström, J., Ilemosoglou, M., Keller, J. A., Vogel, H., & Benedict, C. (2022). Effects of acute sleep loss on leptin, ghrelin, and adiponectin in adults with healthy weight and obesity: A laboratory study. *Obesity, 31*(3). https://doi.org/10.1002/oby.23616

Venuto, T. (n.d.). *How many calories does a pound of muscle burn? Busting the biggest metabolism myth.* Burn the Fat Inner Circle. https://www.burnthefatinnercircle.com/public/How-Many-Calories-Does-A-Pound-Of-Muscle-Burn.cfm

Vogelzangs, N., Kritchevsky, S. B., Beekman, A. T. F., Newman, A. B., Satterfield, S., Simonsick, E. M., Yaffe, K., Harris, T. B., & Penninx, B. W. J. H. (2008). Depressive symptoms and change in abdominal obesity in older persons. *Archives of General Psychiatry, 65*(12), 1386. https://doi.org/10.1001/archpsyc.65.12.1386

Waist size matters. (n.d). Harvard T.H. Chan School of Public Health. https://www.hsph.harvard.edu/obesity-prevention-source/obesity-definition/abdominal-obesity/

Whitaker, K. M., Pereira, M. A., Jacobs, D. R. J., Sidney, S., & Odegaard, A. O. (2017, March). Sedentary behavior, physical activity, and abdominal adipose tissue deposition. *Medicine & Science in Sports & Exercise* 49(3). https://journals.lww.com/acsm-msse/fulltext/2017/03000/sedentary_behavior,_physical_activity,_and.8.aspx

Wigmore, A. (n.d.). *Ann Wigmore quotes.* Goodreads. https://www.goodreads.com/author/quotes/385454.Ann_Wigmore

Wing, R. R., & Phelan, S. (2005). Long-term weight loss maintenance. *The American journal of clinical nutrition*, *82*(1), 222S225S. https://doi.org/10.1093/ajcn/82.1.222s

World Obesity Day 2022 – Accelerating action to stop obesity. (2022, March 4). World Health Organization. https://www.who.int/news/item/04-03-2022-world-obesity-day-2022-accelerating-action-to-stop-obesity

Zbeida, M., Goldsmith, R., Shimony, T., Vardi, H., Naggan, L., & Shahar, D. R. (2014). Mediterranean diet and functional indicators among older adults in non-Mediterranean and Mediterranean countries. *The journal of nutrition, health & aging*, *18*(4), 411–418. https://doi.org/10.1007/s12603-014-0003-9

About the Author

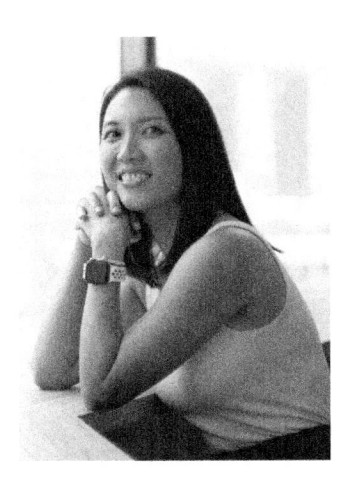

Kelly Kam is a passionate advocate for health and wellness, with a particular focus on weight management. As the well-regarded author of The Belly Fat Prognosis, she has dedicated her life to researching and understanding the complexities of body weight, nutrition, and overall well-being.

Kelly's work is rooted in her belief that everyone deserves to live their healthiest life. She emphasises sustainable methods for maintaining a healthy weight and promotes a holistic approach to wellness that goes beyond mere dieting.

Her book, The Belly Fat Prognosis, provides readers with an understanding of why belly fat accumulates and practical strategies for managing it in the long term.

Readers appreciate Kelly's ability to break down complex health concepts into understandable terms. Her step-by-step guidance empowers individuals to take control of their health journey and make lasting changes.

With her unwavering commitment to promoting health and wellness, Kelly Kam continues to inspire readers with her insightful research and practical advice.

Printed in Great Britain
by Amazon